THE ABC OF
DIABETES

THE ABC OF DIABETES

CARYL DOW JORGENSEN, R.N.,
AND JOHN E. LEWIS, Ph.D.
UK EDITION EDITED BY PETER DAGGETT, M.R.C.P.

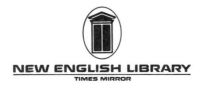

NEW ENGLISH LIBRARY
TIMES MIRROR

Typeset in Palatino by Yale Press Limited, London SE25
Printed and bound in Great Britain by Biddles Ltd,
Guildford and Kings Lynn

ISBN: 0 450 04838 1

Contents

Editor's Preface	6
Introduction	7
How to Use This Book	11
An ABC of Diabetes	15
Appendix A: Abbreviations in Common Use	267
Appendix B: Cookbooks	269
Appendix C: Suggested Reading	270
Appendix D: Emergencies	271
Directory	274
Index	277

Editor's Preface

Caryl Dow Jorgensen and John Lewis have prepared a new kind of manual of diabetes for the interested lay person, an approach which is particularly novel to the United Kingdom where doctors, by tradition, have often explained less to patients than have their colleagues in the United States. My task as editor has been to anglicise their text, without changing the style importantly. The result is a dictionary which will answer nearly all the questions of British diabetics in a language which they will understand, and at the same time provide a little insight into important new developments in the field. Some British doctors will raise points of disagreement, but this is not a bad thing as they will form the basis of helpful discussion with the patient. It cannot be stressed too strongly, however, that the dictionary is only a guide and that it is not a substitute for the advice of a doctor.

Some subjects in the text, such as reference to the various fast food chains, will be ephemeral, while the importance of others, such as ethnic diets, will vary from one part of the country to another. I hope, however, that most of this book will have lasting relevance to all diabetics and that it may settle their doubts and anxieties.

P.R.D.
December 1980

Introduction

The first thing people ask me when they find out I've written a book about diabetes is 'Are you a diabetic?' No, I'm not, but my father was and my mother's father was, and my fourth baby weighed over ten pounds at birth. That makes me diabetes-prone or a 'prediabetic' by most definitions and very interested in diabetes.

I'm also interested in diabetes for professional reasons. Some years ago I worked as a nurse on the Endocrinology Unit at Loma Linda University Hospital, Loma Linda, California. Most of our patients had diabetes, and I was fascinated with the treatment process – listening to the doctors on rounds, the diabetes teaching nurses, the dietitians, and the things the patients had to say.

Diabetes is unique among serious illnesses. It is not curable, but with the proper attention it can be brought under control, so that its effects on the body can be minimised. Moreover, while a doctor must determine the proper course of treatment, its daily maintenance lies largely in the hands of the patient. By regular monitoring of diet, activity, and blood glucose levels, it is seldom difficult to keep diabetes under control. But in order to pay proper attention to these elements, the diabetic must be armed with considerable information. Unaware of this, most people are often extremely upset when they first learn that they have an incurable illness. At the time I was at Loma Linda, I did not realise how difficult it was for the new diabetic to deal with the emotional impact of his disease and at the same time absorb all the information tossed his way by the people involved with his treatment. If it took us professionals years to learn the language of medicine, how could we expect the diabetic to pick it up in a few days or weeks?

After Loma Linda, I worked in other hospitals, which had only poor teaching programmes or none at all. There I tried to do some teaching myself. I was really upset when I read the books and pamphlets that were handed to the patients. As a trained medical professional I could understand the information being offered, but not all the diabetics could. I thought they needed easily accessible material written in non-medical language. Some time later, when I was recovering from a serious automobile accident, and was facing open-heart surgery, I decided to go ahead and write such a book myself. The task, an enormous one, held my life together during a period of great mental and physical stress. My wish is that it will be a help to you and to those around you who care.

The main problem in writing a book like this is that experts do not agree, either on the definition of diabetes, on what tests are best to use to diagnose it, or on the proper treatment. Diabetics even complain that their own doctors don't know enough about the disease. Since I am not a physician, I cannot prescribe; I can only put down facts from books and tapes, and quote doctors and dietitians who have been kind enough to give their permission. It has been almost impossible to use plain English throughout, but where scientific and medical terminology has been necessary, it has been defined as simply as possible.

Dr Charles H. Brinegar, Jr, Assistant Professor of Medicine and diabetologist at Loma Linda University School of Medicine, Loma Linda, California, was very generous in helping me with the initial stages of the book. The assistance of Dr John Lewis, who joined me in completing the manuscript, was of inestimable value. Dr Lewis and I had some real battles over word usage but, by putting ourselves in the place of the reader, I think we have resolved them satisfactorily.

Others who helped were Mary Berry, Librarian, Medical Library, Porterville State Hospital, Porterville, California; Marilyn R. Pankey, Director of Medical Records, Sierra View District Hospital, Porterville, California; Alexander Telesford, MD, Porterville, who saved his medical journals for me. Rowena J. Taylor, BSN, Acting Clinical Director of Porterville State Hospital, and Dr Robert W. Crane, my former personal physician and friend, also of Porterville, both gave help in a time of great stress, and I shall always remember it. I owe a debt I can't pay to my great friend and typist Elna B. Sandeman of Santa Cruz, California. I thank my four children who, though now grown up and scattered, have given me their faith, love, and moral support.

Some of the material in the book will not agree with what is currently taught about diabetes, nor with the way your doctor is treating your diabetes. If you are doing well and you are satisfied with your control, it would probably we unwise to change. If, however, you are not doing well and you are not satisfied, you may want to sit down with him and discuss some new ideas. Failing this, you may wish to seek out a new doctor. We strongly recommend specialists in the treatment of diabetes, realising that these highly trained professionals are not readily available in all areas. Most of all, this book is for you, the person who has diabetes, written with great empathy by two people who know how difficult it is to contend with a body that does not function perfectly.

CARYL DOW JORGENSEN, RN
Sunnyvale, California

My interest in diabetes is both personal and professional. In 1971, the night before I was scheduled to undergo surgery on my knee, I was told I had diabetes. It was difficult to accept the fact that I had an incurable disease. Quite frankly, I refused to accept it at first – I took the fact that I was a diabetic as a personal insult. The next few months were horrible! Trying to walk after the surgery; giving up all the 'goodies' and adjusting the diet; counting calories; using Tes-Tape and insulin. I read all I could on the subject of diabetes. The message gleaned from the reading was simple: It is up to you . . . do not give up . . . it is not that difficult to control. I finally realised I had years of good mileage ahead and I was going to become the master of the situation.

When Caryl Jorgensen asked me to co-author a manual for diabetics, I accepted the invitation with relish. Basic, down-to-earth information on diabetes is lacking. What single reference source can a diabetic turn to in order to find simple basic answers to questions relating to diabetes? Here for the first time was an opportunity to contribute to a manual written in plain English for all to read. (Most diabetics, myself included, fail to take time to know, understand, and educate ourselves about their disease.)

We had some interesting discussions when writing the book, and in the process I learned a great deal. I hope the reader will learn as much about how to care for himself and his disease. We need to be informed.

JOHN E. LEWIS, PHD
Assistant Professor of Medicine and
Pathology
Loma Linda University Medical Center
Loma Linda, California

Professor, Biology
San Bernardino Valley College
San Bernardino, California

1978

How to Use This Book

Our goal in writing this book is to help the diabetic take better care of himself by giving him as much information as possible in non-medical terms. Anyone with a chronic condition such as diabetes lives with it 24 hours a day, and he is the one most responsible for his own care. The doctor plans the treatment for him based on laboratory tests and the information the patient gives him: how the patient feels; the results of home urine tests; any reactions to low blood glucose; and other problems such as infection or slowness in healing, visual disturbances, or symptoms suggestive of blood vessel disease, kidney disease, or damage to the nervous system.

The language of the medical world is a special one, and the lay person must not expect to absorb it in a few hours, days, or weeks. It is not easy to write on a medical subject in non-medical terms, and at times we were forced to use medical terminology. However, in all such instances we have defined the terms; the definitions are included in the alphabetical listings.

This was not planned as a book that one would sit down and read through to learn all about diabetes, but as a reference book. The authors suggest that you take time to read the contents page and the introductions and to browse through the book to get an idea of what we offer you. The subject matter includes a general discussion of diabetes – types, treatment and control. You will find a great deal on diet, food exchanges (both conventional and vegetarian), diet plans, and diets for special situations – illness, exercise, and travel. These you can go over with your doctor, or they can serve as a guide when your doctor is not available. There is information on insulin and other drugs, insulin injections and injection sites, blood and urine tests, the metric system – part of the medical language today – and the problems of day-to-day living with diabetes. A number of longer articles include both general and specific information; specific information may appear as a subhead under the main entry – Insulin Mixtures under Insulin, for instance, or Cholesterol under Blood Tests. In other cases, the reader is referred to other entries for further information; for instance, see Exercise/Sports under Activity. This enables you to read as much – or as little – on any given subject as you wish. How much you get from the book is up to you.

Research in diabetes is big news today. Newspapers and magazines are quick to pick it up. We have included a section on research, and defined many of the words you will see in the news that are associated with research, such as genes, chromosomes, recombinant DNA, and cloning. We hope we have anticipated the trends so that the book will be useful to you over a long period of time.

The
ABC
of
Diabetes

INDEMNITY

This book is not intended as a substitute for medical advice of physicians. The reader should regularly consult a physician in all matters relating to his/her health and particularly in respect of any symptoms which may require diagnosis or medical attention.

A

ABDOMEN The part of the body between the chest and the pelvis. For diabetics the abdomen is an ideal site for insulin injection. See also INSULIN INJECTION AND INSULIN INJECTION SITES.

ABDOMINAL PAIN Pain in the abdomen may be a symptom in diabetic ketoacidosis. It can be severe and described as cramplike. Of course, abdominal pain can be caused by other conditions such as injury or a disorder other than diabetes mellitus. The doctor should be notified if the temperature is elevated and if glucose and/or acetone is present in the urine.

  The doctor will want to know as much as possible about the problem; for example, in addition to pain in the stomach, there may be nausea and vomiting. Diarrhoea may be associated with diabetes and it may occur more at night than during the daytime. See also ACIDOSIS; DIABETIC KETOACIDOSIS: DIABETIC NEUROPATHY: URINE TESTS.

ABLATION Surgical removal of a part of the body.

ABORTION The loss of an embryo or foetus before the fourth month of pregnancy. Diabetic mothers have an abortion rate about 10 to 15 per cent higher than nondiabetics. A spontaneous abortion occurs without medical interference. A therapeutic abortion is performed by a doctor for the well-being of the mother; for example, the mother may have a serious kidney condition that would not allow her to carry a pregnancy to completion without causing a threat to her own life. See also MISCARRIAGES; PREGNANCY AND CHILDBIRTH.

ABRASION Damage to the skin produced by scraping or rubbing in an injury, or by an irritation such as sheetburn. All abrasions should be cleansed with mild soap and water followed by antiseptics, then covered with a sterile dressing. Severe abrasions should be cared for by a doctor or nurse. See also INFECTION AND INFLAMMATION.

ABSCESS A localised collection of pus in any part of the body caused by inflammation or infection.

ABSORPTION OF FOOD The passage of food into the tissues of the body and its use in nourishing the cells of the body.

ACCEPTANCE OF DIABETES MELLITUS See Living with Diabetes under DIABETES MELLITUS.

ACCIDENTS Accidents can be of all kinds and degrees, from a small cut to a serious injury. Do not neglect any injury no matter how small. Keep a first-aid kit at home and in your car. Notify your doctor if the injury is severe, or if you are uncertain about what you should do. Be sure to let him know how you feel; for example, if you are weak or sweaty, if your temperature is elevated, and if you have glucose and/or acetone in your urine. See also INFECTION AND INFLAMMATION: URINE TESTS.

ACETEST See URINE TESTS.

ACETOACETIC ACID See KETONE BODIES; URINE TESTS.

ACETOHEXAMIDE (Dimelor) See ORAL HYPOGLY-CAEMIC AGENTS.

ACETONE See KETONE BODIES; URINE TESTS.

ACETONE BREATH See DIABETIC KETOACIDOSIS; KETONE BODIES.

ACETONURIA Excess acetone in the urine, present during starvation or in diabetic ketoacidosis. See also KETONE BODIES.

ACETYL COENZYME A See KETONE BODIES; KREBS CYCLE.

ACHILLES TENDON The large tendon connecting the muscles of the calf with the heel bone (calcaneus). The Achilles tendon reflex: When the Achilles tendon is struck at the ankle level, the foot normally will extend out and down. In diabetics, this reflex may be lessened or absent altogether. See also DIABETIC NEUROPATHY.

ACID On the pH scale, which measures acidity vs alkalinity, acid reads less than 7. Acids form hydrogen ions when dissolved in water. See also BASE; ELECTROLYTES; pH SCALE.

ACID-BASE BALANCE   The human body is slightly alkaline: 7.35 to 7.45 on the pH scale (anything below 7 is acid, above 7 is alkaline; 7 is neutral). The four main types of acid-base imbalances are (1) metabolic acidosis, (2) respiratory acidosis (3) metabolic alkalosis, and (4) respiratory alkalosis. See also ELECTROLYTES; pH SCALE.

ACIDOSIS   Upset of the acid-base balance in the body. When too many ketone bodies (from the breakdown of fatty acids) or too much lactate (from lactic acid) is produced, the acidity of body tissues and fluids increases and the pH drops below 7.35. The difference in pH is very critical, and the body continually attempts to adjust the pH as it uses food and oxygen throughout the day (the metabolic process). Acidosis can be caused by faulty metabolism, poor control of diabetes, or poisoning. See also DIABETIC KETOACIDOSIS; KETONE BODIES; METABOLIC ACIDOSIS; pH SCALE; RESPIRATORY ACIDOSIS.

ACNE   Inflammation of the fat glands and hair follicles of the skin, specially on the face, chest, and back. These areas often form pustules and cysts with deep skin involvement that may produce scarring. Acne is common during adolescence, and it tends to run in families. In the diabetic it can be a special problem because of the resulting bacterial infections in severe cases. The emotional stress accompanying acne can make diabetes harder to control. A dermatologist (skin specialist) should be consulted for help in treating acne.

ACTIVITY   See EXERCISE/SPORTS (includes a diet for exercise); MANUAL LABOUR.

ACUTE   Sharp, severe – happening fast – as applied either to pain or to disease. Not chronic.

ADDITIVES IN FOOD   See FOOD ADDITIVES.

ADIPOSE TISSUE   Tissue containing fat cells. See WEIGHT.

ADJUNCT   Joined or added to something else. For example, in the treatment of diabetes, when diet alone will not control blood glucose, medication would be an adjunct treatment.

ADOLESCENCE   From the start of puberty to maturity. Puberty is the time of life when boys and girls develop sexually and are able to reproduce. The boy produces sperm and can father a child; the girl begins to menstruate and can bear a child. The average ages in the British Isles for onset of puberty are 13 to 14 for boys and 11 to 14 for girls.

For diabetics, frequent adjustments in insulin dosages and food intake may be necessary during this period of great change. Therefore, if the results of urine tests show an otherwise unaccountable change, either up or down, or weight unaccountably is lost or gained, be sure to contact your doctor.

ADRENAL GLANDS   Two small glands, one each located immediately above each kidney. They consist of two parts, the medulla (inside) and the cortex (outside). The medulla produces the hormones adrenaline and noradrenaline, which are also known as catecholamines; these hormones release glycogen from the liver and muscles as needed and act against the action of insulin (insulin antagonists). The cortex is governed by ACTH (adrenocorticotrophic hormone) from the pituitary gland and produces hormones called steroids, which help maintain the balance of water and mineral salts in the body. The cortex also produces some of the male and female hormones.

A tumour of the adrenal glands, phaeochromocytoma, usually noncancerous, produces extra adrenaline, and can cause high blood pressure. See also ACID-BASE BALANCE; BLOOD PRESSURE; ELECTROLYTES; INSULIN ANTA-GONISTS; PITUITARY GLAND; SODIUM; STEROIDS, STEROLS.

ADRENALINE   See ADRENAL GLANDS.

ADULT   Grown to full size and strength; mature.

ADULT-ONSET DIABETES   See DIABETES MELLITUS, Adult-Onset.

AETIOLOGY   The study of causes; for example, the cause of disease.

AFEBRILE   Without fever; when the body temperature is at its normal level (approximately 98.6° Fahrenheit or 37° Celsius). See also THERMOMETER, CLINICAL.

AGE-HEIGHT-WEIGHT TABLES   See WEIGHT.

AGENT   A substance or force whose action produces change.

AGGRESSIVE BEHAVIOUR   To be aggressive means to attack, either verbally or physically. In the diabetic a change in behaviour may be the first sign of low blood glucose (hypoglycaemia). Since the brain uses glucose primarily for nourishment, lack of available glucose in the blood can cause changes in behaviour, including aggressiveness.

AIR HUNGER The need for oxygen. In diabetic ketoacidosis breathing is laboured, usually deep and gasping. This is known as *Kussmaul's respiration,* named after the German physcian A. Kussmaul (1822-1902) who first described it. See also DIABETIC KETOACIDOSIS.

AIRLINES See TRAVELLING WITH DIABETES.

AIR SICKNESS See TRAVELLING WITH DIABETES.

ALBUMIN One of a group of simple proteins that are soluble in water. Albumin is the major protein in the blood. It is not ordinarily found in the urine; however, in 5 to 11 per cent of normal persons, there is sometimes a small amount of albumin in the urine with no disease present. Albumin in large amounts in the urine is called albuminuria. Diseases in which albumin may be found in the urine and which may related to diabetes are kidney disease, high blood pressure and heart disease. See also BLOOD TESTS; URINE TESTS.

ALCOHOL (Ethanol, or Ethyl Alcohol – Distilled Liquor) Alcohol – distilled liquor – is in a category of dispute; some say flatly that it is a carbohydrate and others that it is an alcohol. It is metabolised (utilised) in the body as a carbohydrate in the Krebs cycle, but yields 7 calories/gram instead of 4 calories/gram as do other carbohydrates. On the food exchange lists it is usually substituted as a fat. All alcohols contain hydroxyl (OH) groups.

Ethyl alcohol is the alcohol found in drinking alcohol such as whisky, gin, rum, vodka, and tequila. An average alcoholic drink has about 100 calories. These calories contain no nutrients and take the place of food in the sense that the alcohol is used as energy before food. Wine and beer do contain some nutrient value. A 12-ounce can of beer contains 145 to 164 calories, 9 to 14 grams of carbohydrate, a small amount of protein, and some minerals; the new light beers have 95 calories, some as low as 70. Dessert wines such as sherry or port are 19 per cent alcohol and contain about 122 calories in each 3 ounces, with 7 grams of carbohydrate. Dry wines – burgundy, chablis, rosé, Rhine wine, and sauterne – are 12 to 13 per cent alcohol, with 4 to 5 grams of carbohydrate. They are more acceptable than sweet wine or beer for use by the diabetic, but they must also be counted as non-nutritive calories. Discuss the use of any alcoholic beverage with your doctor.

Furthermore, alcohol must be considered a drug, and diabetics who take any of the oral hypoglycaemic agents may get a reaction when these drugs are taken in combination with alcohol. This reaction is called a Disulphiram, or Antabuse-like reaction, and usually manifests itself as a flushing or feeling of facial warmth. Other reactions may include headache, difficulty in breathing, nausea, dizziness, or an increased heart rate and pulse. Also, alcohol, especially when taken on an empty stomach, can lower the blood glucose. Large amounts of alcohol taken over an extended period of time may be the main cause of pancreatitis. See also PANCREAS.

ALCOHOL SWABS   To clean the skin before injecting insulin, an ordinary sterile cotton swab soaked in industrial methylated spirit can be used. You can buy the swabs at the pharmacy: store them in a covered jar. Surgical spirit can also be used, however it may cause extra-sensitive skin to become red and irritated. Disposable foil-wrapped alcohol swabs, available from your pharmacy, are more expensive than the dry swabs but are useful away from home. Caution: Keep out of reach of children.

ALIMENTARY CANAL (or Tract)   The digestive system or food tract, over 25 feet long, extending from the mouth through the stomach and intestines to the rectum and anus.

ALIMENTATION   The process of nourishing or feeding the body. This includes chewing, swallowing, digestion, absorption, and use of food by the body.

ALIQUOT   A scientific term designating a definite sample taken from a whole, for example, 6 hours' worth of a 24-hour urine collection, or that part of any collection that is used for actual testing. See also URINE TESTS.

ALKALINE   The opposite of acid. Having the qualities of or pertaining to an alkali, and which, when combined with acid, reacts to make a salt. See also pH SCALE.

ALKALOSIS   Upset of the acid-base balance in the body. See also ACID-BASE BALANCE.

ALLERGENS See ALLERGY.

ALLERGY This is the popular but scientifically outdated term for hypersensitivity of the immediate type. About 10 per cent of the population suffer from allergies of some degree. Some diabetics are allergic to insulin. See INSULIN. Diabetics can also be allergic to other foreign agents that invade the body, such as drugs, pollens, food, insect bites and stings, house dust, and animal dander.

An allergic reaction indicates that the body has been previously exposed to a foreign body called an allergen. When such a reaction occurs, the body manufactures antibodies, a family of proteins produced by certain lymphocytes. Antibodies are also called immunoglobulins. These antibodies combine in a variety of ways in the defence of the individual.

Allergies can be dangerous! Anyone can become allergic to a foreign body at any time in his life. Although it is not common, life-threatening immediate hypersensitivity – known as anaphylactic shock, or anaphylaxis – can cause death in moments by an immediate swelling of the throat and airways in the lungs, shutting off the breath. The symptoms of immediate hypersensitivity occur rapidly (0 to 20 hours) whereas those of delayed hypersensitivity take longer to appear (24 to 72 hours). Reponse to a bee sting, for example, would produce immediate allergic reactions, usually within minutes; the response to a tuberculin skin test is observed after 24 hours. *Never borrow or lend drugs!* If you know you are allergic to something, such as penicillin or bee stings, wear a Medic Alert bracelet or necklace.

Allergies can make diabetes harder to control, because they are stressful to the body. Some drugs given for allergies can cause the blood glucose to rise. This is another reason any doctor treating you should know if you have diabetes. Some drugs for severe allergies are Piriton, an antihistamine, taken by mouth, injection, or infusion directly into the vein, and adrenaline taken subcutaneously like insulin. For some very sensitive persons, the doctor may prescribe one of these drugs to be carried at all times. Fortunately, most allergic reactions are not life-threatening, but may cause only redness of the skin, itching, runny nose, or other little miseries. Any reaction that causes difficulty in breathing (dyspnoea), however, requires an immediate trip to the doctor or to the emergency room of the nearest hospital. See also BITES AND STINGS; BLOOD.

ALPHA CELLS See PANCREAS.

AMERICAN INDIANS and DIABETES See DIABETES MELLITUS (STATISTICS).

AMINO ACIDS Proteins are made of long chains of amino acids. Over twenty kinds of amino acids are known. The body can make all but eight of these, and these eight are called 'essential amino acids'. They are isoleucine, leucine, lysine, methionine, phenylalanine, threonine, tryptophan, and valine. Histidine is also essential for children. When you eat protein, the body breaks it down to amino acids that are used to feed the cells. The body does not store amino acids, but can change them into glucose, which can be stored in the liver and muscles as glycogen, or made into fat. When the body needs energy, the glycogen can be converted back to glucose or to amino acids, although not the eight essential amino acids.

Essential amino acids must come from a diet of first class protein containing all the amino acids, to allow the body to complete protein synthesis (build body tissue). First class protein is found in meats, poultry, fish, eggs, milk, and cheese. Proteins from plants are second class, but a diet containing a variety of plant protein will provide all the amino acids (complete protein). An example of first class plant protein is the Mexican diet combining beans and rice. Breads and cereals that combine several grains will also provide first class protein. A diet containing a wide variety of vegetables, cereals, grains, and legumes is certain to contain all the amino acids. See List 2 and Vegetarian Food Exchanges under FOOD EXCHANGES; PROTEIN.

AMNIOCENTESIS See PREGNANCY AND CHILDBIRTH.

AMNIOTIC FLUID The liquid in the womb that surrounds and protects the foetus (baby) before it is born. See PREGNANCY AND CHILDBIRTH; TOXAEMIA OF PREGNANCY.

AMPULE, or AMPOULE Small, sealed glass bottle or container. It does not have a stopper or cap but is broken open. It is used for sterile preparations intended for injection.

22

AMPUTATION Removal of a limb. In diabetic patients, amputation is usually indicated when gangrene has developed, infection is uncontrolled, pain is excessive, or tissue has been destroyed. Amputation can range from a single toe to an entire limb.

AMYOTROPHY Muscle wasting in the legs caused by nervous system disease: it results in pain, weakness, and weight loss. For unknown reasons, it occurs most often in middle-aged or older men with mild diabetes. Only one leg may be affected at first (asymmetric), but if not controlled, it can affect both legs. The degree of improvement is unpredictable, but with good control of diabetes, keeping the blood glucose levels down, this condition often improves in four to six weeks. See DIABETIC NEUROPATHY.

ANABOLISM See METABOLISM.

ANAEMIA A condition in which either there are not enough red blood cells or the red blood cells do not have enough hemoglobin. There are many causes of anaemia, but chiefly it is associated with an insufficency of iron. The amount of glucose carried by the red blood cells varies with the degree of anaemia; therefore whole blood is seldom used in the measurement of blood glucose, serum or plasma being used instead. See BLOOD.

ANAESTHESIA A partial or complete blockage of sensation with or without loss of consciousness in preparation for a medical or surgical procedure. Under anaesthesia, the diabetic patient should be watched carefully, following the general principles of treatment of diabetes.

ANAESTHESIA – LOSS OF SENSATION This may result from disease of nerves (see PARAESTHESIA) or be temporarily induced by doctors so that operations can be performed. Local anaesthesia is a state of numbness produced by an injection near a nerve (not into it). General anaesthesia is a state of unconsciousness.

ANALGESIC Pain reducing.

ANALYSIS Laboratory tests to determine what substance is present and/or how much. Qualitative analysis identifies the kind of material; quantitative analysis measures the amount of material. See BLOOD TESTS; URINE TESTS.

ANAPHYLACTIC SHOCK; ANAPHYLAXIS See ALLERGY.

ANATOMY The study of the structure of the body, including the bones, blood, muscles, nerves, and internal organs.

ANGER See STRESS.

ANGINA PECTORIS See HEART DISEASE.

ANGIOGRAPHY (Angiogram) A process in which dye is injected into an artery by means of a hollow tube called a catheter to make organs of the body visible. These include the heart, pancreas, and kidneys. The dye is radiopaque (X-rays cannot penetrate it) and allows the doctor to see the condition of the blood vessels on a fluoroscope.

    A fluoroscope is a type of X-ray machine that is turned off and on for short periods of time in order that the target organ can be seen as it functions. Regular X-rays can be taken during angiography, and motion pictures are made for study and diagnosis.

ANHIDROSIS A condition in which sweating or perspiration is absent or is limited to the upper part of the body. Anhidrosis sometimes occurs in the diabetic. People with this condition do not tolerate heat well. See DIABETIC NEUROPATHY; SWEATING.

ANIMAL STARCH See GLYCOGEN.

ANOREXIA Absence or loss of appetite.

ANOXIA A condition in which the blood lacks sufficient oxygen.

ANTABUSE-LIKE REACTION See ALCOHOL; ORAL HYPOGLYCAEMIC AGENTS.

ANTIBIOTICS Chemical compounds (drugs) used to kill micro-organisms (germs) such as bacteria, yeast, and moulds. Some drugs, the sulphonamides, interact with the sulphonylureas and may cause low blood glucose.

    Never take antibiotics unless they have been prescribed by a doctor. Always take them exactly as instructed. If you go to a doctor who has not seen you before, be sure he knows that you have diabetes.

ANTIBODIES See ALLERGY.

ANTIEMETIC A drug that prevents or relieves nausea and vomiting. See TRAVELLING WITH DIABETES.

24

ANTIGENS   See ALLERGY.

ANTIHISTAMINE   See ALLERGY.

ANTIPYRETIC   Any agent that reduces fever. See SALICY-LATES.

ANURIA   Lack of urinary output. See KIDNEYS; KIDNEY DISEASE.

APNOEA   A temporary period when breathing stops.

APOTHECARIES' MEASURE   A system of measuring medicines, now replaced by the metric system. See METRIC SYSTEM.

ARM PAIN   See HEART DISEASE.

ARTERIOGRAPHY   See ANGIOGRAPHY.

ARTERIOSCLEROSIS   See HEART DISEASE.

ARTERY   See BLOOD.

ARTIFICIAL KIDNEY   See HAEMODIALYSIS; RESEARCH.

ARTIFICIAL PANCREAS   See PANCREAS.

ARTIFICIAL SALT   See SODIUM.

ARTIFICIAL SUGARS or SWEETENERS   See SUGAR.

ASCORBIC ACID   Vitamic C. See VITAMINS.

ASEPTIC   Sterile or without living micro-organisms (germs). Aseptic technique is a method by which substances are kept sterile. An example is wiping the top of the insulin vial with alcohol before taking out the insulin and cleaning the skin with alcohol at the site of the injection. Do not touch the needle before injecting – with your fingers or anything else. See INSULIN INJECTION AND INJECTION SITES.

ASPIRATE   To aspirate food means to swallow it the 'wrong way' – through the windpipe (trachea) and into the lungs instead of down the gullet (oesophagus). NOTE: Do not feed a diabetic in a low blood glucose condition if he is having trouble swallowing. See HYPOGLYCAEMIC REACTIONS.

ASPIRATION OF SYRINGE   See INSULIN INJECTION AND INJECTION SITES.

ASPIRIN   See SALICYLATES.

ASYMMETRIC   Occurring on one side only, as on only one side of the body.

ASYMPTOMATIC   Without symptoms.

ATAXIA   Lack of control of movement – to be off balance. This can occur with diabetic ketoacidosis, or with hypoglycaemia, and may be mistaken for drunkenness.

ATHEROMA   A plaque that can clog arteries. See HEART DISEASE.

ATHEROSCLEROSIS   See HEART DISEASE.

ATHLETE'S FOOT   See FEET, CARE OF.

ATHLETICS   See EXERCISE/SPORTS (includes a diet for exercise).

ATROPHY   In a medical context, the wasting away of tissue from disuse or because of improper nourishment, or both.

AUTOIMMUNITY   A condition in which an individual may produce antibodies to his own body tissues. These are called autoantibodies. Autoimmunity plays a role in many situations, including that of ageing, response to infections and other diseases. Specifically related to diabetes, these antibodies may compete with insulin at cell receptor sites. See ALLERGY; CELLS.

AUTOMATIC SYRINGE   See INSULIN SYRINGES AND THEIR CARE.

AUTOMOBILE DRIVING   See DRIVING.

AUTOMOBILE INSURANCE   See DRIVING.

AUTOMOBILE TRIPS   See TRAVELLING WITH DIABETES.

AUTONOMIC NERVOUS SYSTEM (ANS)   See NERVOUS SYSTEM.

AVOIRDUPOIS   A system of measurement in which a pound has 16 ounces and a ton 2,000 pounds (UK = 2,240 pounds). See METRIC SYSTEM.

AZOTAEMIA   See KIDNEY DISEASE.

B

BABIES See FAT BABIES; PREGNANCY AND CHILD-BIRTH.

BACTAEREMIA Bacteria in the blood, popularly called blood poisoning; an infection. See CULTURE.

BACTERIA See MICRO-ORGANISMS.

BACTERICIDE An agent that kills bacteria.

BACTERIURIA Bacteria in the urine, found more often in the diabetic whose blood glucose is not well controlled; some bacteria multiply rapidly in the sugar (glucose) of the diabetic's urine. See also CULTURE; URINE TESTS.

BAKING POWDER, SODIUM-FREE See SODIUM.

BASAL METABOLIC RATE (BMR) With the body at rest, the basal metabolic rate is the smallest amount of energy (or calories) needed to keep the body alive. Activity, high body temperature, infection, anxiety, or other stresses increase the need for food. See METABOLISM; STRESS.

BASE Any substance that will neutralise an acid. See also ACID-BASE BALANCE.

BASEMENT CELL MEMBRANE A membrane consisting of several layers of tissue surrounding the blood capillaries. In the diabetic person, especially when diabetes is poorly controlled, the basement membrane thickens, a condition called microangiopathy, or disease of the small blood vessels; sometimes this condition is the first indication of diabetes. The thickening can cause problems in many parts of the body, especially the eyes and the kidneys. See also BIOPSY; BLOOD VESSEL DISEASE; KIDNEY DISEASE; RESEARCH.

BASIC FOUR FOOD GROUPS See DIET.

BASOPHIL A type of white blood cell. See BLOOD.

BATHING Bathing too often and with too much soap dries the skin and may cause it to crack; this applies to older people and others with dry skin. The old habit of basin-washing is a good one – wash and rinse parts of the body such as under-arms, genitalia, and feet once or twice a day. See also SKIN CARE.

B.D.A. (British Diabetic Association)   See Directory.

BEANS, DRY   See FOOD EXCHANGES, List 4.

BED REST   A person ill in bed will need less food but probably as much or more medication for his diabetes. Individuals taking oral hypoglycaemic agents may need to change to insulin temporarily, because insulin controls the blood glucose better during illness. Those on insulin may need more insulin during sickness. Glucose and acetone test results may be different not only because of sickness, but because bed rest can also change tests. See also BED SORES; CASTS; SKIN CARE.

BED SORES (Decubiti)   Sores caused by pressure from lying in one position too long. A person in bed who is not able to turn alone will need to be turned at least every two hours so that the skin over the bony places, such as the coccyx (end of backbone), heels, toes, and shoulders, does not break down and develop into sores. Bed sores are slow to heal, often requiring additional hospitalisation. For the diabetic they cause extra stress on the body and increase the possibility of infection. To avoid bed sores, keep blood circulating by moving arms and legs frequently. Be sure the sheets are not wrinkled and that the bed is dry and clean – no crumbs, urine or stool. If possible, sit up in a chair several times a day and, if your doctor approves, walk, even if you have to be assisted.

A bed sore starts as a whitened or reddened area that won't massage away. This is caused by a temporary lack of blood and is known as ischaemia. The next stage is usually a blister, which quickly progresses to a sore. Bed sores can start without visible signs by sitting or half sitting for long periods of time. This results in a 'shearing effect', in which layers of tissue beneath the skin are pushed out of position and are deprived of a proper blood supply.

Sheetburn   An abrasion caused by rubbing the skin against the sheets while moving in bed. It usually affects the elbows and the anklebones. It is dangerous for diabetics with feeling-loss, as the skin may be worn away painlessly without the person realising it, which can expose the body to infection. Protect elbows and ankles by wrapping them with gauze or with special protective pads made for this purpose; they are available at hospital supply stores. (See yellow pages of the phone book under Hospital Equipment and Supplies or Physicians and Surgeons Equipment and Supplies).

Alcohol should not be used as a rub because it is so drying to the skin, causing the skin to be extrasensitive and even to crack. Use a good lotion – a doctor or pharmacist will advise you. See SKIN CARE.

BEEF INSULIN   See INSULIN.

BEER   See ALCOHOL.

BEE STINGS   See ALLERGY; BITES AND STINGS.

BENEDICT'S SOLUTION   See URINE TESTS.

BENIGN TUMOUR   See TUMOUR.

BETA CELLS   See PANCREAS.

BETA-HYDROXYBUTYRIC ACID   See KETONE BODIES.

BIGUANIDES   These drugs enhance the peripheral actions of insulin by a mechanism which is not understood completely. Phenformin ('Dibotin') was widely used but is being withdrawn because it can cause lactic acidosis. Metformin ('Glucophage') is an older drug which is less likely to do this. It is made in 500 mg and 850 mg tablets and is taken in a dose of 500 mg to 3,000 mg daily in divided doses. Diarrhoea is sometimes a problem at higher doses.

BI-HORMONAL RESPONSE   Though it is controversial, diabetes mellitus is sometimes referred to as a bi-hormonal, or two-hormone disease, the hormones involved being insulin and glucagon. See GLUCAGON.

BILATERAL   On both sides, such as both sides of the body.

BILE   The liver secretes a solution called bile that is stored in a pear-shaped sac called the gall bladder, where it is concentrated up to twelve times. Even though bile secretion is a continuous process, the flow of bile into the gastro-intestinal tract is not continuous. When food enters the upper part of the small intestine (duodenum), the gall bladder is stimulated to empty the bile into the duodenum. Chemically, bile contains large quantities of bile salts that aid in fat digestion, small amounts of cholesterol, and bilirubin, which is a waste product of red blood cell destruction. The yellowish colour of the skin seen in jaundice is due to bilirubin. See also JAUNDICE; LIPIDS for Cholesterol; LIVER.

BILIRUBIN See BILE; BLOOD.

BINARY FISSION See RESEARCH.

BIOASSAY A method to determine or measure a substance in the body by noting its effect on a live animal or an isolated organ preparation such as cells from the pancreas, liver, or other organs under study *in vitro* (in a test tube).

BIOCHEMICAL Pertaining to the chemistry of living things – all plant and animal life.

BIOPSY The removal of tissue from a living body for examination and testing. In a test to check for thickening of the basement cell membrane, a small piece of muscle tissue (about one millimetre in diameter) is removed with a hollow needle. The muscle tissue is examined under a microscope after special preparation.

BIOSTATOR SYSTEM See RESEARCH.

BIOSYNTHESIS The building (synthesis) of a chemical substance in the normal process that takes place in living cells. This normal process is called the 'physiological' process, as opposed to the abnormal or diseased process. See also PATHOLOGICAL.

BIRTH CONTROL PILLS See CONTRACEPTIVES.

BIRTH DEFECTS See CONGENITAL DEFECTS.

BITES AND STINGS Ant bites and bee and wasp stings can be dangerous to the allergic individual. Clean bites with soap and water; put ice on insect stings. Human bites are usually infected and should be treated by a doctor. If you are allergic to insect stings or bites, your doctor may suggest carrying medication to be taken immediately, either orally or by injection, in the event of a bite or sting.

Family and friends should be informed of the need for prompt attention to severe allergies. WARNING: In the event of an allergic reaction, be sure to notify your doctor that you have diabetes. Some medications used for the treatment of allergies raise the blood glucose. See also ALLERGY.

BLADDER; BLADDER INFECTION See URINARY BLADDER.

BLAND DIET See DIET.

BLEEDING Bleeding from injury, disease, or ulcers is a serious problem; blood loss is stressful to the body and the mental state and can cause complications in the control of diabetes. Open wounds or lesions can also lead to infection, further increasing stress. To control serious visible bleeding, apply a pressure bandage (dressing) by holding the edges of the wound together with tape, if available; then cover with thick layers of any clean fabric (sterile gauze if possible). Tie something around this firmly to hold the dressing taut but not so taut as to shut off the blood supply to an arm or leg. Wounds of the scalp bleed a lot, but are fairly well controlled by a pressure dressing. In the case of serious wounds, call the doctor or go to the nearest hospital. See also HAEMOR-RHAGE; NOSEBLEED.

BLINDNESS Diabetes is the leading cause of adult blindness in the United States; however, only about 2 per cent of diabetics become totally blind. New ways of helping blindness caused by diabetes are being discovered. Good diabetes-control decreases the chance of problems with the eyes, especially if control is started at the time diabetes is first recognised.

Legal Blindness In the United Kingdom, a person is regarded as blind if he or she has insufficient sight for normal employment. In practice this means vision measured as below 6/60, or if there is a major defect in the visual fields. Lesser degress of handicap are described as 'partial sight'. Both 'blindness' and 'partial sightedness' can be registered as disabilities and may entitle the victim to additional social security payments. Diabetes mellitus is the commonest cause of adult onset blindness. See also EYESIGHT; MACU-LA LUTEA; RNIB.

BLISTERS Because of loss of feeling in some diabetics, it is easy for them to get blisters on their hands and feet. These can become infected. To avoid blisters, wear properly fitted shoes with clean stockings. Wash and examine the feet every day. Wear gloves when working with your hands, especially for such activities as gardening or carpentry. See INFECTION AND INFLAMMATION.

BLOOD The life-supporting fluid that circulates throughout the body. The composition of whole blood is both cellular and noncellular (see below). The major function of the blood is to transport oxygen and nutrients to every cell in the body, and to remove from these cells waste products of body function such as carbon dioxide. The three main types of blood cells are red blood cells, white blood cells, and platelets. The noncellular portion of whole blood is called plasma.

Red Blood Cells (also called **Erythrocytes**) Blood gets its red colour from the haemoglobin carried in the red blood cells. Haemoglobin contains iron, carries oxygen from the lungs to the body cells, and carries carbon dioxide as a waste product back to the lungs where it is exhaled into the air. (Oxygen is also exhaled at the same time because the body uses only about 25 to 30 per cent of the oxygen inhaled.)

The normal number of red blood cells in each cubic millimetre of blood is a little more than 5 million in males and a little less in females. The percentage of the blood made up of red blood cells is the haematocrit. The normal per cent is 35 to 45 per cent for females, and 40 to 50 per cent for males, but in anaemic blood it may be much less. Red blood cells are formed in the bone marrow of the adult, and once they enter the circulation, their life span is about 120 days before they disintegrate. The breakdown products are iron, which is transported back to the bone marrow for formation of more haemoglobin, and bilirubin, which is excreted through the liver into the bowel.

White Blood Cells There are five different kinds of white blood cells collectively called leukocytes (an increase in the number leukocytes is leukocytosis; a decrease in the number is leukopenia). Leukocytes are divided into two groups: those containing visible granules in their cytoplasm, the granulocytes, and those without visible granules. See also CELLS.

There are three types of granulocytes. Neutrophils are one type. Composing 60 to 70 per cent of the white blood cells, these police cells move from the blood stream into the tissues to engulf and destroy foreign material such as bacteria. Eosinophils, 1 to 4 per cent of the white cells, are another type. These are usually found in tissues where allergic conditions are developing. In certain diseases, for

32

example, worm infections, the number of eosinophils may increase to 60 per cent or higher. Basophils compose ½ to 1 per cent of the white cells and in the tissue are referred to as mast cells. During allergic reactions mast cells release histamine, which produces runny noses, wheezing, skin rashes, and itching. See also ALLERGY.

There are two types of cells without granules. One type, the monocytes, make up 2 to 6 per cent of the white blood cells and are very effective in destroying foreign materials. Once monocytes leave the blood circulation they become macrophages and, depending on the organ involved, are called liver macrophages, spleen macrophages, or lung macrophages. Lymphocytes, composing 25 to 30 per cent of the white blood cells, are the second type. They are called the 'central cells of the immunologic process' because of the important role they play in defending the body against disease. There are two major populations of lymphocytes, identified as B and T lymphocytes. B lymphocytes synthesise and secrete antibodies (immunoglobulins). T lymphocytes are involved in tissue destruction and hypersensitivity reactions. Both B and T lymphocytes are also found in high numbers in a variety of organs such as lymph nodes, tonsil and adenoids, the appendix, spleen and liver. See also ALLERGY; RESEARCH; THYMUS GLAND.

Platelets (also called **Thrombocytes**) Small fragments of a type of white blood cell formed in the bone marrow. The number of platelets in each cubic millimetre of blood is normally about 400,000. Their function is to aid in blood clotting.

Plasma The fluid portion of blood that contains the blood-clotting protein fibrinogen. If blood is allowed to clot, using the fibrinogen in the formation of the clot, the remaining fluid is called serum. Plasma or serum is used in the laboratory to determine a number of tests that the doctor may need to check in the management of the diabetic. In this light-straw-coloured fluid of the blood can be found sugars, protein, lipids, minerals, salts, hormones, enzymes, antibodies, antigens, and waste products that are transported to and from organs, tissues, and cells of the body. Chemically, plasma or serum can be divided into two major protein components: albumin, which constitutes about 60 per cent, and globulins, which make up the remaining 40 per cent. See also ALBUMIN; ALLERGY; ELECTROLYTES.

Circulation of the Blood   Blood circulation through the blood vessels starts after the left ventricle of the heart has received freshly oxygenated blood from the lungs, by way of the pulmonary vein, which empties into the left atrium and then through the mitral valve and into the left ventricle. The blood is pumped from this chamber through the aorta and the arterial system to small blood vessels called arterioles, which are connected to capillaries. Capillaries are only about one millimetre in length, and large enough in diameter to allow blood cells to travel only in single file. It is during this passage through the capillaries and at no other place that the blood nourishes and otherwise serves the cells of the body.

Small veins called venules connect the capillaries with the blood-returning veins. The whole system is called the vascular system, and together with the heart is referred to as the cardiovascular system. The heart is a pump, forcing blood through the arteries, which themselves are circled by muscles. The return to the heart through the veins is effected by the force of the continuous pumping of more blood. Veins have special valves that keep the blood from falling back; in addition, the action of the muscles of the body as it moves helps squeeze and push blood back to the heart. It is important, therefore, to keep the body as active as possible.

Poor circulation of the blood means the body tissues are not being nourished properly, nor are the waste products taken away as efficiently as required. There are many reasons why circulation may be impaired. Among them are a poor pump (the heart), clogged arteries (atherosclerosis), hardened arteries (arteriosclerosis), lack of exercise, dehydration, and accidents destroy blood vessels. See also BLOOD TESTS; GLUCOSE; HEART DISEASE.

BLOOD COUNT   See BLOOD TESTS.

BLOOD CULTURES   See CULTURE.

BLOOD DYSCRASIA Abnormal condition in the blood caused by poison, disease, and sometimes by reactions to drugs.

BLOOD GLUCOSE   See GLUCOSE.

BLOOD GLUCOSE TESTS   See BLOOD TESTS.

BLOOD INSULIN ASSAY   See Plasma Insulin Levels under BLOOD TESTS.

BLOOD IN URINE (Haematuria)   See KIDNEY; KIDNEY DISEASE.

BLOOD LIPIDS   See LIPIDS.

BLOOD PLASMA   See BLOOD.

BLOOD PRESSURE   The pressure or force of the blood on the walls of the arteries as measured in millimetres of mercury. The average body pressure is commonly set at 120 (systolic) over 80 (diastolic), but there are individual variations within normal limits. A reading of 90/60 may be normal for one person, while 140/80 is normal for another. Blood pressure usually gets higher as one gets older.

Systolic Blood Pressure   The higher blood pressure reading obtained when the heart contracts and pumps the blood through the arteries. The reading measures the force necessary to overcome the resistance of the blood vessels.

Diastolic Blood Pressure   The lower blood pressure reading obtained when the heart is at rest and refilling. It measures the condition of the blood vessels, and it is therefore regarded as the more important of the two readings.

Hypertension, or High Blood Pressure   Hypertension is commonly said to exist when the reading is 150/90 or more, although there is disagreement among doctors over this figure. There are several types of hypertension: (1) primary, or essential, hypertension, in which the cause is not known; (2) secondary hypertension, caused by a known disease such as heart disease or kidney disease (sometimes associated with juvenile-onset diabetes); and (3) systolic hypertension, which shows only high systolic readings and is probably due to arteriosclerosis.

Other suspected causes of high blood pressure are excess body weight and stress – mental or physical (see STRESS). Hypertension can be without symptoms, or it can cause headaches, dizziness, ringing in the ears, or irregular heartbeats.

Hypotension   Low blood pressure.

BLOOD TESTS   There are more than fifty blood chemistry tests; the basic tests related to the usual care of the diabetic are listed here, plus a few more complicated tests. Whole blood, plasma, or serum may be used for tests, depending on the test and the laboratory. Normal adult values are given here, although these may vary slightly from one laboratory to another.

Albumin Serum albumin levels are used to aid in the diagnosis of kidney or liver disease. The normal range is 30 to 50 grams per litre of serum.

Bilirubin Knowledge of the use of bilirubin in the body is necessary in order to understand liver disease. Do not eat yellow vegetables such as carrots or squash before the test; otherwise, there are no food or drink restrictions. Normal total bilirubin levels are less than 17 micromoles per litre. See BILE.

Blood Urea When the kidneys fail to remove urea from the blood, blood urea nitrogen rises. Many factors may contribute to this condition, including dehydration. The normal range is 2 to 7 mmol per litre. See also KIDNEYS; KIDNEY DISEASES.

Complete Blood Count (CBC) Includes red blood cells, platelets, white blood cells, and a white blood cell differential count.

Haemoglobin A Glycosylated haemoglobin. See page 209.

Red Cell Count Normal values range between 4 million and 6 million per cu mm of blood.

Platelet Count Normal values are 150,000 to 450,000 per cu mm of blood.

White Cell Count Normal values are 5,000 to 10,000 per cu mm of blood.

White Cell Differential Count It is often helpful in the diagnosis and treatment of a disease to know the proportion of the five different kinds of white blood cells. The normal range is: neutrophils, 60 to 70 per cent; eosinophils, 1 to 4 per cent; basophils, ½ to 1 per cent; lymphocytes, 25 to 30 per cent; monocytes, 2 to 6 per cent.

Cholesterol No food or drink restrictions unless the test is one to separate different types of cholesterol by electrophoresis. This is not usually done. See also discussion of normal levels under LIPIDS.

Cortisone-Primed Oral Glucose Tolerance Test Cortisone adds an additional stress to the body's ability to produce insulin. This test is designed to diagnose diabetes in the early stages of adult-onset diabetes. Prepare for a test as directed by the doctor. See also DIABETES MELLITUS.

Creatinine Measures kidney function. Normal range is 40 to 120 micromoles per litre of plasma or serum.

Cultures See CULTURE.

Dextrostix (Ames Company) Reagent strips used to test for glucose in the blood. They can be used at home according to the directions on the package by comparing with a colour code on the bottle, or with an Ames Eyetone Reflectance-meter, Dextrometer, Glucocheck or Hypocount. The reading for glucose is more accurate than a urine test, but the sticks are expensive compared with Clinitest tablets for urine testing. The Eyetone machine is very expensive, and requires a doctor's prescription to purchase. The test requires sticking a finger or earlobe with a sterile needle or lance. Constant use makes the fingertips sore. The machine is used in emergency rooms, some doctors' offices, and special hospital units. See also RESEARCH; URINE TESTS.

Electrolytes The electrolytes most often measured are potassium (K), sodium (Na), chloride (Cl), and bicarbonate (HCO_3). The normal range is potassium, 3.5 to 5 millimoles per litre (mmol/L); sodium 138 to 145 mEq; chloride, 95 to 106 mEq; and bicarbonate, 22 to 26 mEq. See also ELECTRO-LYTES.

Fasting Blood Sugar or Fasting Blood Glucose (FBS or FBG) This test is done in the laboratory using plasma or serum. Depending on who interprets the test, values of 6.7 mmol/L or more of plasma or serum are diagnostic of diabetes. Two tests are done on separate occasions. Do not eat after midnight; however, you may drink plain water.

Glucose Tolerance Test (GTT) See Oral Glucose Tolerance Test (below).

Glycemie 20/800 Reagent strip for measuring blood sugar without a meter.

Haematocrit, or Packed Cell Volume (PCV) This test measures the relative volume of red blood cells and plasma in the blood. Normal range is 40 to 50 per cent for males and 35 to 45 per cent for females.

Haemoglobin A test to measure the amount of red oxygen-carrying material (haemoglobin) in red blood cells. Normal range is 12 to 16 g/dl for females and 14 to 18 g/dl for males.

Insulin Levels See PLASMA INSULIN LEVELS.

Oral Glucose Tolerance Test (OGTT) Also called **Glucose Tolerance Test (GTT)** This is a test of the body's ability to handle glucose. For three days before the test the diet should include a fixed amount of carbohydrate, from 150 to 300 grams, depending on the doctor's order. Patients on a reducing diet may be told to eat 150 to 300 grams of carbohydrates for five to seven days before the test. No food is eaten after midnight on the day before the test. On the day of the test, urine and blood samples are first collected for the fasting state; then the patient is given a flavoured drink containing a measured amount of glucose. Patients are advised to sit during the test. The test may last from 2 to 5 hours, depending on the doctor's order.

After the fasting blood and urine are taken, urine is usually collected after ½ hour, 1 hour, 2 hours, and at the 3rd, 4th and 5th hours, if a longer test is done. A blood sample will also be drawn at these times. You may feel weak, nervous, or sweaty (a hypoglycaemic reaction). Be sure to let the laboratory personnel know if you have these symptoms or feel sick.

Intake of water during the test is encouraged, but nothing else, not even chewing gum. Smoking is not permitted.

Preparation for test: No food after midnight, but drink water so you can produce urine for the tests.

Though the oral glucose tolerance test is still being used to diagnose diabetes, many authorities feel that this test is too stressful to the body and are replacing it with the fasting blood glucose test.

Packed Cell Volume (PCV) See test for haematocrit (above).

pH Measures acidity or alkalinity in the blood. No food or drink restrictions. Normal range is 7.35 to 7.45.

Plasma Glucose See tests for fasting blood sugar (glucose) (above) and random blood sugar (glucose) (below).

Postprandial   See Two-Hour Postprandial Test (below).

Random Blood Sugar (RBS) or Random Blood Glucose (RBG)   Measures the amount of glucose in the blood at a given time. No food or drink restrictions.

Triglycerides   A test for blood lipids. The doctor may order a special diet. There is a 12 to 14-hour fast before the test. Normal range is 1.4 to 8.3 mmol/L of serum. See also LIPIDS.

Two-Hour Postprandial Test (2-hr PP)   This is a test for glucose in the blood. Two hours after the meal, blood is drawn. Postprandial means 'after a meal', but instead of a breakfast high in concentrated carbohydrates, the doctor may give you a measured amount of glucose in a flavoured drink. Blood is then drawn two hours after the last swallow. The plasma glucose should be 6.7 mmol/L or below at 2 hours.

White Blood Cells   See test for complete blood count (above).

BLOOD UREA   See BLOOD TESTS.

BLOOD VESSEL DISEASE   There are two types of blood vessel diseases: macroangiopathy, more prevalent in adult-onset diabetes, affecting the large blood vessels of the body which include the heart, the brain, and the periphery – particularly the feet; and microangiopathy, more prevalent in juvenile-onset diabetes, affecting the small blood vessels, particularly those of the kidneys and the retina of the eye.

The blood vessels leading to and serving the brain may be affected, causing strokes. See also CEREBROVASCULAR ACCIDENTS.

Doctors feel there is a relationship between high blood glucose and blood vessel disease. Lipids in the blood can also increase blood vessel disease causing atherosclerosis. See also HEART DISEASE; LIPIDS.

BLOOD VESSELS   See BLOOD.

BLURRED VISION   See EYESIGHT; RETINA, RETINO-PATHY.

BODY IMAGE   See Living with Diabetes under DIABETES MELLITUS.

BODY TEMPERATURE   See THERMOMETER, CLINICAL.

BOILS   Inflammations or infections in the subcutaneous layer of the skin, glands, or hair follicles. Boils are more common in uncontrolled diabetes. See also INFECTION AND INFLAMMATION; SKIN CARE.

BORDERLINE DIABETIC See Classification of Diabetes under DIABETES MELLITUS.

BOVINE INSULIN Insulin prepared from the pancreases of cattle. See also INSULIN.

BOWELS The intestines. See CONSTIPATION; DIABETIC NEUROPATHY; DIARRHOEA.

BOWMAN'S CAPSULE See KIDNEYS.

BP British Pharmacopoeia. An official list of approved drugs, under their chemical names. The list contains a description of each drug; the letters BP after a drug indicate that it is on the list. Commercial drug manufacturers call their products by a 'trade' name. For example, chlorpropamide is sold under the trade name Diabinese.

BPC British Pharmaceutical Codex. A more extensive list of widely used drugs.

BRAIN The brain uses primarily glucose for food, but when glucose is not available, it can also use ketone bodies, which are converted to glucose. It is very important to avoid a condition of low blood glucose (hypoglycaemic reaction) because the brain may be damaged when no glucose is available.

BRAND NAME See TRADE NAME.

BREAD EXCHANGES See FOOD EXCHANGES, List 4.

BREAKFAST See DIET; FOOD EXCHANGES.

BREAST FEEDING See PREGNANCY AND CHILDBIRTH.

BREATHING In hypoglycaemia or low blood glucose, breathing can become fast and shallow. In hyperglycaemia or high blood glucose, diabetic ketoacidosis can cause air hunger, in which breathing becomes deep and gasping and is known as Kussmaul's respirations. The breath may smell fruity from acetone, and the face may be red. Both symptoms are serious, and though low blood glucose (hypoglycaemia) usually can be treated at home, diabetic ketoacidosis must be treated in the hospital. See also ACETONE BREATH; AIR HUNGER; HYPOGLYCAEMIC REACTION.

BREATH ODOUR See ACETONE BREATH; MOUTH CARE.

BRIGHT'S DISEASE Nephritis, or inflammation of the kidney. See also KIDNEYS; KIDNEY DISEASE.

BRITISH DIABETIC ASSOCIATION See Directory.

BRITTLE DIABETES See DIABETES MELLITUS.

BUNIONS See FEET, CARE OF.

BURNS A diabetic who has lost some sense of feeling (anaesthesia) should be careful when using electric appliances, hot tap water, heating pads, and hot-water bottles and when smoking cigarettes. A water temperature of 110°F (43.3°C) or less is considered safe. Be sure heating pads are used on the lowest heat setting; wrap hot-water bottles well in heavy towels. Over-exposure to the sun is always a danger because it damages the skin. Diabetics who take oral hypoglycaemic agents may be subject to photosensitivity and receive severe sunburn. This can be very stressful, causing problems with control of the blood glucose.

BUS TRIPS See TRAVELLING WITH DIABETES.

BUTTER Butter has the same number of calories as regular margarine – about 45 per teaspoon, or 5 grams of fat – and is equal to one fat exchange. A pat of butter served in restaurants has 100 calories and 11 grams of fat. Because butter is a highly saturated fat, margarine made from polyunsaturated fats is a better choice for those who have to limit their fat intake. See also FOOD EXCHANGES, List 6; MARGARINE.

C

CACHEXIA Serious malnutrition.

CAESAREAN SECTION See PREGNANCY AND CHILDBIRTH.

CAFFEINE A drug in the xanthine group obtained commercially from tea. Caffeine is a stimulant to the nervous system, causing the adrenal glands to secrete adrenaline which raises the blood glucose by causing the liver to convert glycogen to glucose. It also increases the flow of acid to the stomach, and is thought to contribute to blood vessel and heart disease in some people.

There are 100 to 150 mg of caffeine in a cup of brewed tea or coffee, with a trace in cocoa. Most of the caffeine is removed from decaffeinated coffee. The amount in cola and other soft drinks varies.

CALCIFICATION The process by which tissues become hardened by a deposit of mineral salts, as in, for example, the arteries. One of the causes of arteriosclerosis. See also BLOOD VESSEL DISEASE; HEART DISEASE.

CALCULATING A DIABETIC DIET See DIET.

CALLUSES See FEET, CARE OF.

CALORIE The amount of heat it takes to raise the temperature of 1 kilogram of water 1 degree Celsius. This is the large Calorie, of Kilocalorie, written with a capital C, which is 1,000 times larger than the small calorie used in physics. In speaking of food, whether the large or small C is used, it is understood that Kilocalorie is meant. When measured, 1 gram of protein yields 4 calories; 1 gram of carbohydrate yields 4 calories; 1 gram of fat yields 9 calories; 1 gram of alcohol (distilled liquor) yields 7 calories. When food is eaten it produces heat and energy, which are also measured in calories. See also DIET; EXERCISE/SPORTS; FOOD EXCHANGES.

CAMPS There are many summer camps run especially for diabetic children. They are staffed by people with special training to care for the children's needs. The children receive a great deal of education along with the regular camp activities. Summer camp is a good opportunity for an uncertain diabetic child to experience how other diabetic children cope with their problems. Contact the British Diabetic Association for the names of nearby camps.

CANCER OF THE PANCREAS See PANCREAS; TUMOURS.

CANDIDA ALBICANS A fungus infection in the yeast group, also known as candidiasis, moniliasis, and thrush. The most common sites of Candida infection are the mucous membranes of the mouth and genital tract. Suspicion of diabetes may be aroused by the presence of a severe infection causing irritation, severe itching, and sometimes in the female a chronic discharge. See also GENITALIA; MICRO-ORGANISMS; URINARY BLADDER.

CAPILLARIES See BLOOD.

CAPSULE A small gelatine container that is used to package a dose of medicine. The capsule dissolves in the stomach and releases the medicine.

CARBOHYDRATES Sugars and starches. Diabetics must be careful about eating carbohydrates because they are broken down by the body to glucose (blood sugar). Glucose travels in the blood to the liver and muscles where it is stored as glycogen to be released into the blood when the body needs food and energy. Carbohydrates yield 4 calories/gram.

Sugars – which are concentrated carbohydrates – are ordinarily used very quickly in the body, but they are not handled easily by the diabetic because of the lack of available or effective insulin. Long-acting carbohydrates, such as the starches (grains, potatoes, many vegetables, rice, lentils, and beans), are used more slowly in the body and can be used in the diet of the diabetic. It was formerly recommended that calories derived from carbohydrates constitute 40 to 50 per cent of the diet; however, many doctors and nutritionists are now raising this to 50 to 60 per cent. Your doctor or dietitian will give you a diet that will be calculated for the amount of carbohydrate you are to eat. If you are overweight, it will be a reducing diet; if you are active and still growing, you may need to eat more of everything, including carbohydrates. See also DIET; FOOD EX-CHANGES; POLYSACCHARIDES; SUGAR.

CARBON An element. One of the atoms found in food and body tissue.

CARBONATED DRINKS See CAFFEINE; SOFT DRINKS.

CARBON DIOXIDE (CO$_2$) A by-product of reactions (metabolism) that take place in the cells. Animals, including humans, exhale large quantities of CO$_2$ from the lungs. Plants use CO$_2$ as a starting material in the production of carbohydrate materials that animals then use for fuel. See also KREBS CYCLE; METABOLISM.

CARBUNCLE Skin infection composed of a cluster of boils.

CARCINOGENIC Tending to cause cancer.

CARCINOMA Cancerous growth or tumour. See TUMOURS.

CARDIAC DISEASE See BLOOD VESSEL DISEASE; HEART DISEASE.

CARDIOLOGIST A specalist who treats diseases of the heart.

CARDIOVASCULAR SYSTEM The system of the heart and the blood vessels. See also BLOOD VESSEL DISEASE; HEART DISEASE.

CARE OF SYRINGES See INSULIN SYRINGES AND THEIR CARE.

CAR TRIPS See TRAVELLING WITH DIABETES.

CASTS Injury to the body may require a plaster cast. The cast must fit so that the blood can circulate properly. Signs that a cast is too tight are pain, coldness or numbness, a change in skin colour from the normal colour to a bluish or purplish hue. Lack of circulation can also open the door to infection, of which a bad odour can be one sign. Sniff around the edges of a cast or get someone to do it for you to detect the odour of possible infection. Injury with or without infection is a stress to the body that produces an increase in blood glucose. Keep records of glucose and acetone; an increase in medication may be necessary for a time.

CASTS – IN URINE Crystals that may be suggestive of kidney disease or a change of drug therapy.

CATABOLISM See METABOLISM.

CATALYST A substance that produces a change without itself undergoing a change. See also ENZYMES.

CATARACT   See EYESIGHT.

CATECHOLAMINES   See ADRENAL GLANDS.

CATHETER; CATHETERISATION   A catheter is flexible rubber or plastic tube that is inserted into various parts of the body.. Its function is to drain body fluids, or to infuse fluids or drugs into the body, including radiopaque dyes required for angiograms. The most common kind of catheter is the urinary catheter that is placed into the bladder to drain the urine. A Foley catheter is one that is left in the bladder for an indefinite period.

CELLS   The basic biological unit of all living things except viruses. Plants and animals are composed of millions of cells, and are called multicellular organisms, whereas bacteria, yeasts, and other micro-organisms are single-celled and are therefore referred to as unicellular organisms. Plant cells have a rigid outer cell wall protecting the cell membrane and its contents; animal cells lack the cell wall but they are surrounded by a cell membrane. Within the cell two distinct areas can be found: the cytoplasm and the nucleus.

Cytoplasm   The part of the cell that is outside the nucleus but contained within the cell membrane. The living cell appears granular when viewed under a microscope, but actually it is very high in water content (intracellular water) and has a highly active environment, rich in internal bodies. Most of the chemical activities within the cell take place in the cytoplasm. An example of this is protein (enzyme) synthesis.

Nucleus   A distinct area, usually surrounded by a nuclear membrane, containing the nucleic acids deoxyribonucleic acid (DNA) and ribonucleic acid (RNA). The basic function of DNA is the control of cell activity and heredity. It stores all the information necessary to construct and operate life systems. DNA is composed of a long double strand of nucleic acids, while RNA is usually a single strand that acts as a messenger (mRNA) carrying information from DNA to the cytoplasm. In the cytoplasm, in conjunction with other RNA molecules, enzymes are formed.

Chromosomes   The building blocks of DNA – *chromo* means colour and *some* means body; they can be coloured with certain dyes so that they can be seen when viewed through a microscope. Structurally they are long, coiled, springlike bodies composed of nucleotide units. Each plant or animal species is normally characterised by the number of chromosomes in the nucleus of its cells. Humans have forty-six, including the two called X and Y that determine the sex of the individual (two Xs, XX, in the female, and the XY combination in the male).

Genes Distinct units of DNA on the chromosomes. They store all genetic information for protein (enzyme) synthesis and heredity. Gene locus is a term used to designate the section of a chromosome occupied by a gene. Recessive genes are those that are masked by a stronger or more dominant gene.

Receptor Sites Insulin receptors are areas on the surface of the cell's membrane that 'recognise' the hormone insulin. After insulin attaches to the receptor it induces changes in the membrane; these changes set in motion the intracellular processes that stimulate cellular uptake of glucose and the conversion of glucose to glycogen in liver and muscle. Evidence suggests that chemically the receptors are glycolipids, amino acid chains with short chains of sugar and fat molecules attached at various points along their length. It has been estimated that an average fat cell has some 10,000 such receptors. See also RESEARCH for a discussion of cell cloning and recombinant DNA; BLOOD for a discussion of red blood cells and white blood cells; HEREDITY.

CELSIUS (C) Replaces centigrade as the name of the metric system measuring temperature.

CENTIMETRE (cm) See METRIC SYSTEM.

CENTRAL NERVOUS SYSTEM (CNS) See NERVOUS SYSTEM.

CENTRAL VENOUS PRESSURE (CVP) The pressure of the blood in the vein close to the right upper chamber (atrium) of the heart. To measure CVP a small plastic tube or catheter is inserted into a vein and manoeuvred into position. This catheter is part of a closed system including an intravenous infusion that serves as fluid for a measuring gauge (manometer) at the bedside. As ordered by the doctor, or as needed, a reading is made periodically to give an idea of the amount of blood circulating throughout the body. Since severe fluid loss (dehydration) occurs in many patients who are seriously ill – especially in diabetic ketoacidosis and hyperglycaemic hyperosmolar nonketotic coma – it is important that a CVP line be inserted to monitor blood volume. Hypovolaemia is blood volume below normal, and hypervolaemia is blood volume above normal.

CEREALS   See FOOD EXCHANGES, List 4.

CEREBROSPINAL FLUID (CSF)   Protective and supportive fluid surrounding the brain and spinal cord. It consists of water, protein, glucose, urea, and salts.

CEREBROVASCULAR ACCIDENT (CVA)   A stroke. A condition in the brain in which the blood supply is affected, damaging or causing tissue death. The patient may recover completely, partly, or die.

High blood pressure and blood vessel disease are common in poorly controlled diabetes, and contribute to the danger of strokes.

CHANGE OF LIFE   See MENOPAUSE.

CHARCOT JOINTS   Bone changes, usually in the feet and ankles, which can be caused by nervous system disease associated with diabetes. There is usually little pain; instead, there is numbness, stiffness, or tingling complaints (polyneuropathy). Not much can be done beyond applying a cast or performing surgery to make the patient more comfortable. Keeping blood glucose levels in good control can often prevent this rare and little understood form of diabetic neuropathy. See also DIABETIC NEUROPATHY.

CHEESE   See FOOD EXCHANGES, List 5.

CHEMICAL BONDS   When one atom or element combines with another, it does so by means of a number of different bonds or connections. When one molecule of glucose joins with another molecule of glucose, a chemical bond holds them together.

CHEMICAL DIABETES   See Classification of Diabetes under DIABETES MELLITUS.

CHEMICAL NAME   Generic name (of a drug). See page 112.

CHEMICAL PRESERVATIVES   See FOOD ADDITIVES.

CHEMOTHERAPEUTIC AGENT   A medicine or drug that helps the body fight infection or disease.

CHEST PAIN See HEART DISEASE.

CHEWING TOBACCO See TOBACCO.

CHILDBIRTH AND CHILDREN See PREGNANCY AND CHILDBIRTH.

CHILDHOOD DIABETES See DIABETES MELLITUS, JUVENILE-ONSET; PREGNANCY AND CHILDBIRTH.

CHIROPODIST See FEET, CARE OF.

CHLORPROPAMIDE Diabinese. See ORAL HYPOGLYCAEMIC AGENTS.

CHOCOLATE Made from the bean of the cacao or cocoa tree, it has more fat than cocoa. Chocolate is full of sugar. Half a regular-size chocolate bar can be eaten in the event of a hypoglycaemic reaction (which see). See also COCOA.

CHOLESTEROL See BLOOD TESTS; LIPIDS.

CHOLESTEROLAEMIA Cholesterol in the blood. See also BLOOD TESTS; LIPIDS.

CHROMIUM A mineral found in the body in very small amounts (.006 grams). It is involved in the metabolism (use by the body) of glucose. Available in a balanced diet, it is found in fats, vegetable oils, meats, grains, and brewer's yeast. For individuals who have a deficiency of chromium, chromium supplements may help to improve the metabolism of glucose; but such supplements do not seem to have any effect on glucose metabolism where there is no deficiency of chromium in the body.

CHROMOSOMES See CELLS.

CHRONIC Lasting a long time. Opposite of acute, it usually applies to pain or disease.

CIRCULATION OF THE BLOOD See BLOOD.

CIRCUMCISION Removal of the foreskin of the penis. See also GENITALIA.

CITRIC ACID CYCLE See KREBS CYCLE.

CLASSIFICATION OF DIABETES See DIABETES MELLITUS; PREGNANCY AND CHILDBIRTH.

CLAUDICATION See LEG PAIN.

CLEAN CATCH URINE SPECIMEN See CULTURE; URINE TESTS.

CLEAR INSULIN Soluble insulin. See INSULIN.

CLEAR LIQUID DIET See DIET.

CLINIC A place where one may get professional medical or nursing help and advice. Public health departments and hospitals may have special clinics for all kinds of health problems, mental and physical

CLINICAL Referring to the symptoms and the course of a disease as observed by a doctor and other health professionals.

CLINICAL NURSE SPECIALIST See NURSES.

CLINICAL THERMOMETER See THERMOMETER, CLINICAL.

CLINISTIX See URINE TESTS.

CLINITEST REAGENT TABLETS AND COLOUR CHART See URINE TESTS.

CLONES See RESEARCH.

COCOA Made from the bean of the cacao or chocolate tree. The amount of fat varies up to 23 per cent. Cocoa also contains a small amount of caffeine.

COFFEE See CAFFEINE.

COLD FEET See FEET, CARE OF.

COMA A state of unconsciousness that is reached through stages called 'levels of consciousness', as follows: (1) the drowsy patient who can be reached by speech or touch, but who usually responds only by mumbling or with jerky body movements; (2) the patient is stuporous – responding only to moderately painful stimuli, such as pinching of the skin; (3) deep stupor in which the patient responds only to very painful stimuli, such as the pressing of one's thumbnail hard against the patient's sternum (breastbone) or thumbnail; and (4) coma, in which the patient makes no response whatsoever.

Coma can occur with severe injury and disease, including diabetes. Diabetic ketoacidosis, hyperglycaemic hyperosmolar nonketotic coma, lactic acidosis, and severe low blood glucose (hypoglycaemia) can each progress to coma. Of these, coma resulting from low blood glucose presents the most urgent medical emergency because of possible damage to brain cells. When there is a question as to which type of coma exists, treatment for low blood glucose is always begun first.

COMBINING INSULINS See Insulin Mixtures under INSULIN.

COMPLEX SUGARS   See POLYSACCHARIDES.

COMPLICATIONS OF DIABETES   See DIABETES MELLITUS.

COMPOUND FATS   See LIPIDS.

CONCENTRATED CARBOHYDRATES   See SUGAR.

CONDENSED MILK   An evaporated milk containing sugar. Do not confuse condensed milk with plain evaporated milk, which has only had some of the water removed and contains no extra sugar.

CONDIMENTS   Spices, herbs, and relishes. Many condiments have no food value, but relishes and ketchup usually contain sugar and should be avoided. Consult cookbooks for diabetics for recipes for making sugar- or salt-free recipes of all kinds. See also FOOD FLAVOURINGS.

CONFINEMENT   The time during which a baby is born. See also PREGNANCY AND CHILDBIRTH.

CONFUSION   For diabetics: if you are confused, 'muddled' – forgetting what you were doing or saying a moment before – it could mean that your blood glucose is low. See also HYPOGLYCAEMIC REACTIONS.

CONGENITAL DEFECTS   Birth deformities or defects – whether hereditary or the result of illness or injury at time of birth. The congenital defects in children of diabetic mothers are about 13 per cent as compared to 6 per cent in the nondiabetic population. The children of diabetic fathers do not seem to have any more congenital defects than those of nondiabetic mothers, however.

CONGESTIVE HEART FAILURE   See HEART DISEASE.

CONSTANT CARBOHYDRATE DIET   See DIET.

CONSTIPATION   Difficult or delayed emptying of the bowel. It may be caused by damage to the nervous system – diabetic neuropathy – affecting the peristaltic action of the muscles surrounding the bowel. Large amounts of faeces may collect, a condition called faecal impaction. (On the other hand, diabetic neuropathy may produce diarrhoea in some people.) See LAXATIVES.

CONTRACEPTIVES   Oral contraceptives, or birth control pills, containing oestrogens are not generally used in diabetes or, when used, only with close supervision by a doctor. Oestrogens tend to raise the level of blood glucose and can raise blood pressure. No contraceptive is 100 per cent effective except sterilisation.

Mechanical Contraceptives.

1. Intrauterine device (IUD): A plastic or metal device which comes in several shapes; it is inserted into the uterus by a doctor. It is thought to prevent pregnancy by keeping the fertilised egg from attaching to the tissues of the uterus. It may be left in place until such time as pregnancy is desired, or for a maximum of five years, at which point a doctor can remove it; a new one can be inserted after a brief resting period. Examination by a doctor is necessary at least once a year, or any time the IUD causes pain or extra discharge from the vagina.

2. Condoms, or 'rubbers' which fit over an erect penis to collect the ejaculated sperm and prevent it from entering the vagina. Discard after use. May be bought without prescription at a pharmacy.

3. Diaphragm: A flexible rubber dish-shaped device inserted into the vagina over the end of the cervix, the bottom tip of the uterus. The initial fitting is made by a doctor. It is most effective when spread with spermicidal jelly or foam before insertion, which helps prevent sperm from entering the uterus. A diaphragm must be left in place for eight hours after sexual intercourse, after which it is removed, cleansed with warm water and mild soap, and dried.

4. Voluntary sterilisation: For the male there is vasectomy, a surgical procedure in which a piece of the duct (vas deferens) carrying sperm is cut out and the ends tied off, preventing the passage of sperm to the penis. Female sterilisation is effected by a tubal ligation, in which the Fallopian tubes are cut and tied to prevent the sperm from reaching the ovum (egg). This is done by surgical approach though the abdominal wall.

Contact FPA for further information. See FPA.

CONTRAINDICATION   A reason for not giving some types of drugs; for example, a known allergy (hypersensitivity) to a drug means it should not be given.

CONTRAST MATERIAL   See RADIOPAQUE DYE.

CONTROL OF DIABETES   See DIABETES MELLITUS.

CONVULSION See SEIZURES.

COOKBOOKS FOR DIABETICS Most of these cookbooks include instructions on how to use the exchange system and how to weigh and measure food. Many of them are available at local bookstores and libraries or through an interlibrary loan. Ask the librarian for help.†

COOKING Baking, steaming, broiling, and barbecuing are the best ways to cook food. If the food is boiled, do not use too much water or save the water for soups (refrigerate or freeze the stock until needed). Food can be fried using a fat exchange (see FOOD EXCHANGES). Avoid food fried in deep fat.

CORNS See FEET, CARE OF.

CORN SYRUP A syrup of glucose (dextrose) and maltose made from corn. See also SUGAR.

CORONARY See HEART DISEASE.

CORONARY BYPASS SURGERY See HEART DISEASE.

CORTISONE; CORTISOL (HYDROCORTISONE) Hormones made in the adrenal glands. There are insulin antagonists working against insulin and thus raise the blood glucose. See also BLOOD TESTS.

COTTON WOOD EXUDATES See RETINA, RETINOPATHY.

COXSACKIE B A virus. See MICRO-ORGANISMS; RESEARCH.

CRAMPS See ABDOMINAL PAIN; LEG PAIN.

CRANIAL NERVES See NERVOUS SYSTEM.

CREATINE Creatine is a synthesis product of three amino acids present in animal tissue. When it is used by the body (metabolised), it produces creatinine, an end product, which is normally excreted in urine in small amounts. See also Creatinine Clearance Test, under URINE TESTS.

CREATININE CLEARANCE TEST See URINE TESTS.

CREATININE TEST See BLOOD TESTS.

CRYOPEXY See RETINA, RETINOPATHY.

CRYSTALLINE ZINC INSULIN Soluble insulin. See INSULIN.

CUBIC CENTIMETRE (cc) See METRIC SYSTEM.

†See Appendix B: Cookbooks

CULTURE   A laboratory test to determine whether or not micro-organisms are present in the body, and if so, what kind. Samples of blood or urine, exudates from a wound, and sputum are among materials used for culture. The material is placed on special bacteria-breeding material in a dish and placed in an incubator for 24 hours or more. Any growth is examined under a microscope for identification. It is then further tested to determine the best antibiotic to use in treating the infection. See also MICRO-ORGANISMS; URINE TESTS.

CUTANEOUS   Referring to the skin. See also SKIN CARE.

CYCLAMATES   See Sugar Substitutes under SUGAR.

CYSTITIS   An inflammation or infection of the urinary bladder. Symptoms of a bladder infection are painful bladder spasms, the feeling of a need to urinate frequently, and burning sensations in the meatus as the bladder empties. See also CANDIDA ALBICANS; CULTURE.

CYSTOGRAM   A test in which radiopaque dye is inserted in the bladder by means of a catheter. The outline of the bladder can then be seen by X-ray.

CYTOPLASM   The part of a cell that is not the nucleus. See also CELLS.

D

DEAD SPACE See INSULIN SYRINGES AND THEIR CARE.

DEAFNESS See HEARING LOSS.

DEATH RATE OF DIABETICS See DIABETICS MELLITUS, STATISTICS.

DEBRIDEMENT Clearing out the dead tissue from a wound, usually with surgical instruments.

DECAFFEINATED COFFEE See CAFFEINE.

DECILITRE (dl) See GLUCOSE; METRIC SYSTEM.

DECUBITI (S. decubitus) See BED SORES.

DEFENCE MECHANISMS AGAINST DISEASE See ALLERGY; LYMPH, LYMPHATIC SYSTEM; White Blood Cells under BLOOD.

DEFENCE MECHANISMS – PSYCHOLOGICAL See DIABETES MELLITUS, LIVING WITH DIABETES.

DEGENERATION; DEGENERATIVE The deterioration or breakdown of any part of the body due to injury or disease; pathological. In diabetes this is largely due to blood vessel disease in which the blood supply to a part is decreased or cut off completely.

DEHYDRATED FOOD Food that has had the water removed from it. Add water according to directions on the package and use the food the same as any other food. Dehydrated food has the same number of calories as fresh food, and is a satisfactory nutritional source.

DEHYDRATION Loss of water in the body. In the diabetic this occurs in diabetic ketoacidosis, lactic acidosis, and hyperglycaemic hyperosmolar nonketotic coma. It can also occur in one who has a high fever, severe vomiting, diarrhoea, and who has not replaced lost fluids. Some of the symptoms are dry tongue, soft eyeballs (which feel softer to the touch through the eyelid than normal), and 'tenting' a condition in which the skin when pinched up gently makes a tentlike fold and remains that way for a short period of time.

DELIVERY OF A BABY   See PREGNANCY AND CHILD-
   BIRTH.
DELTA CELLS   See PANCREAS.
DEMOGRAPHICS   See DIABETES STATISTICS.
DENTAL CARE; DENTURES   See MOUTH CARE.
DEOXYRIBONUCLEIC ACID (DNA)   See CELLS.
DEPRESSION   A state of low mental and physical energy
   that can be stressful to the system. Blood glucose levels may
   be affected, increasing because of decreased activity or
   increased food intake, or decreasing if food intake is de-
   creased. A person who is severely depressed may not have
   the energy to make urine tests, and may even forget to take
   insulin or other drugs. It is very difficult to deal with severe
   depression. If it cannot be handled at home, hospitalisation
   may be required. See also Living with Diabetes under
   DIABETES MELLITUS; STRESS.
DERIVED LIPIDS   See LIPIDS.
DERMATITIS   See SKIN CARE.
DERMATOLOGIST   A medical doctor who treats diseases
   and conditions of the skin.
DERMATOPHYTOSIS   Athlete's foot. See FEET, CARE OF.
DERMOPATHY   See SKIN DISEASES.
DESICCANT   A tablet or small packet of a chemical that
   absorbs water and keeps drugs and reagent strips dry. Do
   not remove desiccants from the bottle as long as there are
   tablets or strips remaining to be used.
DETACHED RETINA   See RETINA, RETINOPATHY.
DEXTROSE   See GLUCOSE.
DEXTROSOL   A pure glucose sweet which dissolves very
   quickly in the mouth and which is suitable for treating
   hypoglycaemia. One sweet contains about 5 grams of glu-
   cose.
DEXTROSTIX   See BLOOD TESTS; RESEARCH.
DIABETES, ACCEPTANCE OF   See Living with Diabetes
   under DIABETES MELLITUS.
DIABETES ASSOCIATIONS   See BRITISH DIABETIC ASSO-
   CIATION (BDA)*; International Diabetes Federation (IDF)

*See Directory

under TRAVELLING WITH DIABETES: JUVENILE DIABETES FOUNDATION (JDF).

DIABETES CAMPS   See CAMPS.

DIABETES DIAGNOSIS   See DIABETES MELLITUS.

DIABETES IN CHILDREN   See DIABETES MELLITUS, JUVENILE-ONSET.

DIABETES COMPLICATIONS   See BLOOD VESSEL DISEASE; DIABETIC NEUROPATHY; KIDNEY DISEASE; KIDNEYS; RETINA, RETINOPATHY.

DIABETES INSIPIDUS   The term *insipidus* is of Latin origin and means 'tasteless', for in contrast to the urine of persons with diabetes mellitus, who have sweet-tasting urine, those with diabetes insipidus do not have sugar in their urine. Diabetes insipidus is a rather rare metabolic disease; it occurs when the posterior (rear) lobe of the pituitary gland fails to produce sufficient antidiuretic hormone (ADH), a hormone that conserves water in the body. Diabetes insipidus may occur as a primary disease – a congenital defect – usually in male children, or as a secondary disease when the posterior pituitary lobe is destroyed. The net result in both primary and secondary diabetes insipidus is a deficit or absolute lack of ADH, resulting in the daily loss of tremendous quantities of water through the kidneys in the form of urine. The treatment is with drugs that inhibit water loss. Diabetes insipidus is not related to diabetes mellitus.

DIABETES MELLITUS   The term is derived from two Greek words meaning 'to go through or siphon' and 'honey'. What goes through is urine – sweet urine containing glucose (sugar). This is the origin of the old name of diabetes, 'sugar diabetes', in contrast to the tasteless urine of diabetes inspidius described in the preceding entry. For the purposes of this book, the word 'diabetes' means diabetes mellitus.

Diabetes was originally thought to be one disease or condition, but it is now generally accepted to be a condition that has more than one cause, and is probably more than one disease. This is why it has been so difficult to define diabetes. The Joslin Clinic in Boston defines diabetes as a lack of effective insulin.

Diabetes occurs either as a primary disease of unknown

cause or as a secondary disease caused by loss or damage to pancreatic tissue or by the excess of hormones that work against insulin (see INSULIN ANTAGONISTS). Among these antagonistic hormones are some of the adrenal hormones, growth hormone, and glucagon. Obesity is also an insulin antagonist; certain drugs such as birth control pills may trigger diabetes in susceptible persons; and pregnancy and other stresses to the body, both mental and physical, can cause diabetes to show recognisable symptoms in the person predisposed to the disease. Diabetes caused by drugs and pregnancy may be reversible. See also PREGNANCY AND CHILDBIRTH.

Primary diabetes includes two categories: growth- or juvenile-onset diabetes, and maturity-, late-, or adult-onset diabetes.

Diabetes Mellitus, Juvenile-Onset   In this type of diabetes – also known as ketosis-prone – no effective insulin is produced. The category includes diabetics 15 years of age or younger, although the diagnosis of juvenile-onset diabetes is sometimes not made until much later in life. The age at which juvenile-onset diabetes is most likely to be diagnosed is during the growth and prepuberty years, ages 10 to 12. The onset of juvenile-onset diabetes is often quite dramatic; the child can become ill (and look ill) within the space of a few weeks, or even days. Since the blood glucose is high, the osmotic pressure in the blood is high, drawing fluid out of the tissues (see OSMOSIS). A large amount of urine is produced (polyuria) accompanied by great thirst (polydipsia), and, because so much glucose and therefore so many calories are being lost in the urine, the child eats a great amount of food and still loses weight. He will need to urinate day and night and, if he is very young, he may wet the bed. He may be very irritable – unlike his usual self – and display great fatigue and lassitude. Lastly, he may not heal well when he is cut, and infections may occur where previously there was no problem. The diagnosis is rather easy to make in the presence of these overt symptoms.

The juvenile-onset diabetic needs treatment, information, support, and reassurance. Treatment consists of insulin injections once or twice a day as prescribed by a doctor, an appropriate diet, and exercise. Books and pamphlets are available through doctors, drug companies, libraries, book stores, and at camps for diabetic children. The British Diabetic Association (BDA) can provide advice to diabetic children and their parents. Their journal *Balance* contains a children's section.

The juvenile-onset diabetic, because he gets diabetes earlier in life, has diabetes longer on the average than the adult-onset diabetic. Complications of juvenile-onset diabetes tend to be those of the small blood vessels (microangiopathy) affecting the kidneys and the retina of the eye. See RESEARCH for a report on some of the work in progress dealing with control and treatment of diabetes.

Diabetes Mellitus, Adult-Onset This type of diabetes may be called ketosis-resistant, nonketotic, or mild diabetes. Most diabetics, perhaps more than 80 per cent, are in this group. Adult-onset diabetes is most often diagnosed in persons aged 40 or over who are usually obese and could probably be controlled by weight loss and diet alone. Those who cannot control their diabetes by diet alone require oral hypoglycaemic agents and may eventually need insulin. The diagnosis of this type of diabetes is more difficult to make, because the onset is often slow and deceptive. It may be discovered only when other problems take the patient to the doctor, such as trouble with vision, heart disease, pain, numbness and tingling (especially in the legs and feet), and fatigue and headache. Gum problems may prompt an alert dentist to send his patient to a physician, who may then examine him and make a diagnosis of diabetes.

People speak of 'borderline diabetics', which is a confusing and unscientific term, since either one has diabetes or doesn't have it – just as one cannot be only a little bit pregnant. Better terms are 'latent', 'diabetes-prone', or 'prediabetic'.

Treatment of Diabetes Diabetes should be treated as any other disease is treated. The doctor decides what he is treating, knows what he expects to happen, and will know when that goal is reached. See DIABETOLOGIST.

Classification of Diabetes Diabetes has been divided into stages. (See PREGNANCY AND CHILDBIRTH for the Classification of Diabetes of the pregnant female.) The characteristics of each stage have been adapted here from a number of sources: (1) prediabetics, which includes those who are genetically predisposed to diabetes but show no signs or symptoms of the disease, even with diagnostic testing; (2) *chemical* diabetes, sometimes called subclinical or latent diabetes, in which individuals show no signs or symptoms, have a normal fasting blood glucose, but have abnormal results on stress testing such as the oral glucose tolerance test; and (3) *overt* diabetes in which the clinical diagnosis is made on the basis of symptoms and abnormal test results. This classification may change during the next few years, as our knowledge of diabetes increases. See also BLOOD TESTS.

Cure and Prevention   There is no cure for diabetes, unless researchers can learn to replace defective pancreatic beta cells, or to implant artificial pancreases (see RESEARCH). Can overt diabetes be prevented in the person who is by definition a prediabetic? At this point, it is probably not possible to give an answer to that question, for if one is predisposed to diabetes genetically, lives long enough, and is sufficiently stressed, diabetes is most likely to become clinically apparent. There are choices to make: to keep body weight at ideal levels or below, to eat little or no concentrated cabohydrates (sugar), to exercise regularly, and to avoid severe mental or physical stress. In particular, a woman must consider carefully the number of children she wants to bear, as pregnancy is diabetogenic.

Control of Diabetes   This involves accepting the fact that you have an incurable, chronic disease, which is discussed in the following section. There are a few basic rules: Do not skip meals; do not eat more at one meal to make up for eating less at another; eat at the same times; stick to your diet; and exercise regularly. See also DIET; EXERCISE/SPORTS (includes diet for exercise); FOOD EXCHANGES.

Living with Diabetes   This means first that you must fully accept the fact that you have a chronic disease that is incurable at this time. Both authors of this manual live with incurable chronic diseases; we know what a shock it is to learn that you have such a disease. There is a period of adjustment in which you actually mourn the loss of your normal, healthy, invulnerable body. You may become very angry, either with yourself, or with your family, or with the doctor who had to tell you. Or you may become depressed and feel that life isn't worth living. There is nothing more maddening than to have someone say, 'Cheer up! It could be worse!'; or 'You could be killed crossing the street!' Others mean well but they don't understand the terror, anger, and despair you may feel inside.

Parents of young children with diabetes may feel guilty – that perhaps their child's illness is their fault, the result of neglect or improper care. (See HEREDITY.) As the child grows older and learns to assume more responsibility for his own treatment, diet control, and giving his own injections, he may feel he is different from other children. Well, he is. He has diabetes, and must assume more responsibility for his own behaviour at an early age, but he can be taught to control diabetes and not to let diabetes control him. More strict control of blood glucose may mean that the juvenile diabetic will develop fewer of the severe complications of diabetes, or that he will have milder forms of the complications. Also, today there is better understanding of diet and the importance of exercise.

The adult with mild diabetes has fewer actual problems, but he may not believe this. He still may feel that the end of the world has come. He should not depend for help on 'old hands' – people who have had diabetes for a long time; research at the University of North Carolina, reported by Patricia Lawrence, RN, shows that it is the old hands who make the most mistakes. Join the BDA, and the local groups as recommended by your doctor.

The best thing a person with a chronic disease can have is a family that is on his side, accepting, loving, and supporting. But not all families or all members of families can accept the illness of another, and may be less able to deal with it than the one who is sick. Diabetics who live alone may arrange for friends and neighbours to call. In some areas nurses from the National Health Service and district nurse services make calls. See NURSES.

Learn all you can about diabetes, its control, and what

to do if you are ill. You have to make a lot of decisions on your own, for your doctor isn't with you all the time. You have diabetes 24 hours a day, 365 days a year and *no one* can be expected to be there all the time. You spend most of the time alone with your problem. Do not use diabetes to try to get your own way or to avoid living a full and normal life. See also GAMES DIABETICS PLAY.

Lastly, choose a doctor you can trust – one with whom you feel comfortable – one who really knows how to treat diabetes. Most doctors who are qualified to treat diabetes are specialists in internal medicine (internists), endocrinologists, or diabetologists. Since doctors are people, some you will like and have confidence in, and some you will not. You are not being disloyal if you change doctors – you are only cheating yourself if you don't find one who will fit your needs.

DIABETES MELLITUS (STATISTICS) Diabetes, as generally defined occurs in about 1 per cent of the population of the United Kingdom. Surveys to detect the disease, however, suggest that another 1 per cent of the population have the condition, but are unaware of it. The true number (prevalence) of diabetics is therefore likely to be nearer 2 per cent of the population in the Western countries. It is much higher in some groups, notably in the Pima Indian tribe of North America. Diabetes runs in families and this applies both to the juvenile-onset and maturity-onset types. It may soon become possible to identify patients at risk of developing the disease, so that a careful watch can be kept for the first symptoms.

DIABETES PILL See ORAL HYPOGLYCAEMIC AGENTS; RESEARCH.

DIABETES PUBLICATIONS See APPENDIX B: COOKBOOKS; APPENDIX C: SUGGESTED READING; and BIBLIOGRAPHY, at the back of this book.

DIABETES RESEARCH See RESEARCH.

DIABETES SUMMER CAMPS See CAMPS.

DIABETES TEACHING NURSES See NURSES.

DIABETES TESTS See BLOOD TESTS; URINE TESTS.

DIABETES, TRAVELLING WITH See TRAVELLING WITH DIABETES.

DIABETIC ACIDOSIS See COMA; DIABETIC KETO-
ACIDOSIS; LACTIC ACIDOSIS.

DIABETIC DERMOPATHY See SKIN DISEASE.

DIABETIC DIET See DIET; EXERCISE/SPORTS; FOOD EX-
CHANGES; TRAVELLING WITH DIABETES.

DIABETIC FOODS These are not necessarily the same as
dietetic foods. See DIABETIC DIET (above); DIETETIC
FOODS.

DIABETIC KETOACIDOSIS Diabetic ketoacidosis is the
most common type of metabolic acidosis, with high blood
glucose, large amounts of ketone bodies in the blood, and
large amounts of ketone bodies in the blood and the urine. It
is rare today, because the education and treatment of the
diabetic is improving. But ignorance is still the major contri-
buting factor in the occurrence of ketoacidosis. For instance,
there may be errors in medication in the ketosis-prone
diabetic – too little insulin or too much food, or both; neglect
of illness, infection, injury, or other stress; or surgery in the
presence of unrecognised diabetes. The usual laboratory
tests – fasting blood sugar (glucose), complete blood count,
differential count, haematocrit, urinalysis, and electrolytes
(see BLOOD TESTS; URINE TESTS) – do not necessarily
show the presence of diabetes.

*It cannot be emphasised enough that any diabetic, mild or
severe type, can become a victim of ketoacidosis if sufficiently
stressed and neglected – either by himself or his family or in his
medical treatment.*

The symptoms of ketoacidosis first show up as an
increase in blood glucose, followed by increased glucose
and ketone bodies in the urine, which is measured as
acetone in home tests. The onset is usually slow, a matter of
days, but it can happen in a matter of hours. Increased
glucose in the blood causes a shift in water, or an osmotic
diuresis (see OSMOSIS), in which electrolytes are lost,
especially potassium and sodium. Great thirst with large
amounts of urine results in dehydration. The potassium loss
affects the rhythm of the heart and may produce an irregular
pulse. Additional symptoms are abdominal pain similar to
acute appendicitis, nausea with or without vomiting, and
weight loss. As the patient becomes more and more acido-

tic, there my be confusion leading to coma. The treatment is immediate hospitalisation to lower the blood glucose and to reverse the acidosis. See also ACIDOSIS; COMA; HYPER-GLYCAEMIC HYPEROSMOLAR NONKETOTIC COMA; LACTIC ACIDOSIS; METABOLIC ACIDOSIS.

DIABETIC LIPAEMIA Fat or fatlike substances in the blood accompanied by severe glucose intolerance. See also LIPIDS.

DIABETIC NEUROPATHY Disease of the nervous system. Nerve fibres serve all parts of the body, so in theory an injury or disease to any nerve can affect any part of the body. Though diabetic neuropathies are probably the most common complaint in the complications of diabetes, they are not well understood. Recent investigation indicates that high blood glucose over a long period of time is damaging to nerve cells. Some of this damage can be reversed with the lowering of blood glucose to normal levels.

Diabetic neuropathies are divided into two categories: (1) somatic and (2) visceral.

Somatic, or peripheral, neuropathy is the most common, and involves the nerves of the lower legs. Report numbness, tingling, and leg pain to your doctor. See FEET, CARE OF.

Visceral neuropathy may affect any organ or system in the body. It is important to report to the doctor any dizziness or problem with vision, hearing (although this is rare), swallowing, digestion, or elimination of body wastes from the bladder or the bowel. The male may experience retrograde ejaculation or sexual impotence. See also CON-STIPATION; DIARRHOEA; GASTROINTESTINAL TRACT; IMPOTENCE; LEG PAIN; RETROGRADE EJACULATION; SEXUAL INTERCOURSE; URINARY BLADDER.

DIABETIC RECIPES See APPENDIX B: COOKBOOKS. See also DIET.

DIABETOGENIC Tending to cause diabetes. Certain drugs may raise the blood glucose and so may certain conditions, such as pregnancy and childbirth, virus infections, obesity, and a family history of diabetes. Be sure your doctor knows all the drugs you are taking, even vitamins and those drugs you buy over the counter. *Do not borrow or lend drugs to* *friends*. See also HEREDITY; RESEARCH.

DIABETOLOGIST   A doctor who specialises in diabetes. However, most diabetologists are specialists in internal medicine (internists) or endocrinologists. See also Living with Diabetes under DIABETES MELLITUS.

DIABINESE   See ORAL HYPOGLYCAEMIC AGENTS.

DIAGNOSIS   From a Greek word meaning 'to discern'. A medical diagnosis identifies the patient's disease or condition.

DIALYSIS   See discussion of peritoneal dialysis and haemodialysis under KIDNEY DISEASE.

DIAPHORESIS   Abnormal sweating, as when drops of sweat pour out of the skin and run off in streams, causing water loss (dehydration).

DIARRHOEA   Loose, watery stools. The causes may be infection (such as dysentery), nervousness, disease, nerve damage, or poor diabetic control. Severe diarrhoea produces dehydration and loss of electrolytes. When it is caused by nervous system disease, it may occur off and on, often at night, giving it the name 'nocturnal diarrhoea'. If the diarrhoea causes severe electrolyte loss, dehydration, or a rise in body temperature, it can make the control of diabetes more difficult. Check your urine for glucose and acetone; take your temperature and call your doctor. See also DIABETIC NEUROPATHY.

DIASTIX   See URINE TESTS.

DIASTOLIC   See BLOOD PRESSURE.

DIET   People tend to think of the word 'diet' as referring to a special purpose: a reducing diet, a low-fat or low-sodium diet, a diabetic diet, a vegetarian diet, and so on. A diet, however, simply means the food one eats. Basically, a diabetic diet is a diet that would be good for almost anyone! All diets should be formed around the basic four food groups: (1) milk, cheese, and other milk products; (2) meat, fish, poultry, eggs, legumes, dry beans, peas, and nuts; (3) vegetables and fruit; (4) breads and cereals. CAUTION: These are not food exchanges; they are sources of nutrients, and everyone should eat some of the foods from each group every day – preferably with each meal, except for snacks.

Diet Therapy   The treatment of a disease or condition, all or in part, by diet. It is a customary procedure in the treatment of diabetes, either alone or along with oral hypoglycaemic agents or insulin. (Dr Leo P. Krall of the Joslin Clinic in Boston and Harvard University, has said that diet is the best oral hypoglycaemic agent there is.) If the diabetic is over-weight, the diet will be designed to reduce weight and to maintain weight loss. Exercise is also important in the treatment of diabetes; for a diet for exercise, see EXERCISE/ SPORTS. Your doctor will prescribe a diet for you just as he prescribes a drug for your needs.

Since diets are based on the basic four food groups listed above, all diets are a combination of carbohydrates, proteins, and fats. There is disagreement regarding the percentage of calories that should be provided by each of these categories. In the past, it was generally felt that diabetics could not handle carbohydrates in large amounts; thus, their carbohydrate intake was limited, and most of their calories were supplied from protein and fat. Although they are not conclusive, studies now show that diabetics handle long-acting carbohydrates (starches) adequately, and many diabetic diets are now being designed to include 50 to 60 per cent of the daily caloric needs from carbohydrates, 15 to 20 per cent from protein, and 20 to 30 per cent from fats. A more usual diet would derive 40 to 45 per cent of its calories from carbohydrate, the difference being made up with protein and fat. Sugars are quick-acting carbohydrates, and though small amounts of sugar can be included in the diabetic diet from time to time sugar raises the levels of blood glucose rapidly, leads to obesity in many persons, causes tooth decay, and should generally be avoided by all heath-conscious individuals.

Calculating a Diabetic Diet To determine the number of grams to eat of each type of food, multiply the recom-mended total number of calories by the per cent recom-mended for each category, and divide by the number of calories per gram for that particular category. For example, in a 1,500-calorie diet based on 60 per cent carbohydrate, 20 per cent protein, and 20 per cent fat, the following computa-tion would be used:

CARBOHYDRATE

$$\frac{.60 \times 1500}{100 \times 4} = \frac{900 \text{ calories}}{4 \text{ calories/gram carbohydrate}} = 225 \text{ grams carbohydrate.}$$

PROTEIN

$$\frac{.20 \times 1500}{100 \times 4} = \frac{300 \text{ calories}}{4 \text{ calories/gram protein}} = 75 \text{ grams protein.}$$

FAT

$$\frac{.20 \times 1500}{100 \times 9} = \frac{300 \text{ calories}}{9 \text{ calories/gram fat}} = 33 \text{ grams fat.}$$

This means that a diet using 225 grams carbohydrate, 75 grams protein, and 33 grams fat would satisfy a 1,500-calorie daily allowance. For examples of a 1,500-calorie diet with snacks, see FOOD EXCHANGES. You can use the Food Exchange system or a diet given to you by your doctor, or you can experiment with your own diet provided you discuss this with your doctor.

Remember to spread the intake of all foods, including carbohydrates, over the entire day. Your doctor or dietitian will discuss with you the best way for you to spread the total calories throughout the day – 4, 5, or 6 meals, counting snacks. The division will depend to some extent on your work and life-style. It will help your doctor if you keep good records of what you eat, what activity you engage in, and urine tests for glucose and acetone. Two methods of dividing the total number of calories throughout the day are as follows:

4 MEALS	6 MEALS
2/7 breakfast	4/18 breakfast
2/7 lunch	2/18 midmorning snack
2/7 supper	5/18 noon
1/7 bedtime	1/18 3 hours after lunch
	5/18 supper
	1/18 bedtime

Young diabetics need food for growth as well as energy. This is sometimes managed by the constant carbohydrate diet, in which the number of calories from carbohydrates remains the same from day to day, but proteins and fats may be eaten freely. This diet might also be suitable for certain very active, lean, adult diabetics who maintain normal weight. If your doctor approves this type of diet, he will determine the number of calories you will need from carbohydrates. To adapt this, see the Food Exchange lists that give both the calories and grams. Regular lists of food giving only calories can be changed to grams by dividing the number of calories by 4. In this case we are talking only about carbohydrates – there is no limit on protein or fat.

Free diet A basic, nutritious diet, in which calories and concentrated carbohydrates (sugars) are restricted.

Soft Diet Easy to chew, easy to digest, and without any harsh fibre, roughage, or rich or spicy foods. May be used in the presence of infection or following surgery.

Clear Liquid Diet Water, clear broth, thin gruels made with water, plain gelatine, tea, and coffee. This diet varies from doctor to doctor and from hospital to hospital and may include carbonated beverages. It is used for a limited period of time, 24 to 36 hours, because it is nutritively poor.

Full Liquid Diet Strained fruit juices, strained or blended gruels, strained creamed soup, ice cream, gelatine, junket, custard, tea, coffee, milk, cocoa. It is usually prescribed for the post-operative patient or the acutely ill patient.

Meal Planning – General Hints Eat all meals on time every day in order to keep the blood glucose levels as normal as possible. Each meal should include the proper balance of carbohydrates, proteins, and fats. It is a good idea to plan menus ahead of time with this in mind, and to plan grocery shopping so that the right foods are available at home.

Learn to understand the Food Exchange lists. See also DIET SCALE.

For a discussion of eating out in restaurants, homes of friends, while travelling, see TRAVELLING WITH DIABETES; for *fast-food restaurants* (such as McDonald's and Kentucky Fried Chicken), see FOOD EXCHANGES; for diets for sick days, see SICKNESS; for diets for exercising, see EXERCISE/SPORTS; ethnic diets, see FOOD EXCHANGES; for low-sodium diets, see SODIUM.

DIETETIC FOOD Food for special diets, but do not confuse 'dietetic' with 'diabetic'. Dietetic foods may be low in sodium, or fat, or sugar, but they still contain calories that must be counted in the diet. Diabetics should be made fully aware of this, and usually will be advised to eat regular food that can be prepared at home without sugar, or with sugar substitutes. Food Exchanges are based on regular food. Diet soft drinks or tonic are generally acceptable. Discuss dietetic foods with the dietitian or doctor.

Diet mayonnaise and diet margarine are often exceptions to the use of dietetic food, particularly for those on a low-fat diet. Diet margarine contains about 50 per cent water; 2 teaspoons are one fat exchange (see FOOD EXCHANGES, List 6).

DIET FOR EXERCISE See EXERCISE/SPORTS.

DIET FOR SICKNESS See SICKNESS.

DIETITIAN See REGISTERED DIETITIAN.

DIET PILLS Do not take any diet pills unless they are ordered by your doctor.

DIET SCALE If the food exchange system of diet is used, a good diet scale that indicates grams (see METRIC SYSTEM) as well as ounces and weighs items up to 25 pounds will be needed. If you cook in quantity, weigh the ingredients as they are added, keeping a total calorie count. After cooking, divide into servings, and calculate the number of calories per serving by dividing the total number of calories by the number of servings. Bread, soup, stews, casseroles, and other food can be cooked this way and stored in the refrigerator or freezer. Mark the containers giving the number of calories and servings.

DIET THERAPY See DIET.

DIFFERENTIAL COUNT A white blood-cell count giving the percentages of the various kinds of white blood-cells present in the blood. This is useful in diagnosis of infection and disease. It is part of a complete blood count (CBC). See also BLOOD TESTS.

DIGESTION After food is eaten, it is broken down in the

stomach and intestines to a form that the body can use. Carbohydrates (starches and sugars) are broken down to glucose; proteins and amino acids; and fats to fatty acids and glycerol. Amino acids and fatty acids can be converted to glucose by the body and can then be used for energy, repair of tissues, replacement of cells, and storage as glycogen and fat. In the process, digestive juices, enzymes, and some hormones, including insulin, are used. See also GLUCOSE POTENTIAL OF FOODS.

DIGESTIVE TRACT   See ALIMENTARY CANAL.

DIMELOR   See ORAL HYPOGLYCAEMIC AGENTS.

DIM VISION   See EYESIGHT.

DINING OUT   See TRAVELLING WITH DIABETES.

DIPLOPIA   See EYESIGHT.

DISABILITY BENEFITS   See SOCIAL SECURITY.

DISACCHARIDES   Double sugars. See SUGAR.

DISPOSABLE SYRINGES   See INSULIN SYRINGES AND THEIR CARE.

DISULPHIRAM REACTION   See ALCOHOL.

DIURESIS; DIURETICS   Diuresis is a condition in which more than the usual amount of urine (polyuria) is produced. It can be caused by diabetes, among other conditions, and by drinking too much liquid (polydipsia). It can be induced by diuretics, commonly known as 'water pills'. In addition to the pill form, taken by mouth, diuretics can be injected intramuscularly or intravenously. They aid the body in getting rid of excess fluid (found in heart and kidney disease) and are also used to lower blood pressure.

High blood glucose acts as a powerful osmotic (see OSMOSIS) diuretic in diabetic ketoacidosis and hyperglycaemic hyperosmolar nonketotic coma.

DIVIDED DOSES OF INSULIN   See INSULIN.

DIZZINESS   A condition that may be a symptom of low blood glucose, nerve damage to the inner ear, or other conditions.

DOMINANT GENES   See CELLS.

DNA   Deoxyribonucleic Acid. See CELLS.

DOUBLE VISION   Diplopia – seeing things double. See EYESIGHT.

DOUBLE-VOIDED URINE SPECIMEN   Same as second-voided urine specimen. See URINE TESTS.

DRAM   A fluid measurement in the apothecaries' system of measurement. A dram is a scant teaspoon or 4 to 5 cc. See APOTHECARIES' MEASURE; METRIC SYSTEM.

DRIED FOOD   See DEHYDRATED FOOD.

DRINKING ALCOHOL   See ALCOHOL.

DRIVING   It is generally felt that diabetics in good control have no problem and can truthfully answer 'no' to a question regarding physical disability on a licence application. Many feel it is a matter of personal conscience, while others think a doctor should certify whether an individual is able to drive safely. If the diabetes is not in good control, the doctor may not give certification to drive. Do not drive a car on an empty stomach; allow time for snacks or regular meals for a long trip. Keep dextrose sweets (Dextrosol) in a car, purse, or pocket regularly; carry identification as a diabetic; pull over to the side of the road if you feel any symptoms of low blood sugar; and *never drink alcohol before or during driving.* Stop and walk around every hour or so on long trips to aid circulation. See TRAVELLING WITH DIABETES.

Automobile Insurance   If you have insurance and discover you have diabetes, the best advice seems to be to stay with the same company. New policies for diabetics are judged on an individual basis. There is usually no trouble getting insurance if diabetes is under control, but do not hide the fact that you have diabetes; the insurance company might be reluctant to pay. In addition, it may not be possible to get a personal accident income policy clause if insulin is being used. See also INSURANCE.

DROPSY   See OEDEMA.

DROWSINESS   This may be a danger signal: a sign of hypoglycaemic reaction, and the first stage in a descending level of consciousness. Eating a piece of fruit can help raise the blood glucose level. See COMA; HYPOGLYCAEMIC REACTIONS.

DRUG INHIBITION   See INHIBITION.

DRUG INTERACTION   When two or more drugs are taken together, the action of one may change or interfere with the action of another. Alcohol is a drug and, in combination with oral hypoglycaemic agents or insulin, it can cause low blood glucose, especially if it is taken on an empty stomach. Be sure the doctor knows all the drugs you are taking, including non-prescription drugs.

DRUG OVERDOSE A reaction of the body to excess amounts of a drug. Too much insulin or oral hypoglycaemic agents can result in a lowering of the blood glucose. The same effect is achieved if too little food is eaten while regular doses of these drugs are taken. An overdose of other drugs will probably affect the diabetes medication. An overdose of some drugs can result in coma and death. If a change in behaviour is observed and there is reason to suspect an overdose, call a doctor immediately, or take the patient to the nearest hosptial.

DRUG POTENTIATION See POTENTIATION.

DRUG SENSITIVITY When you are taking a drug or medication, especially if you have not taken it before, advise the doctor if you experience nausea, diarrhoea, a skin rash, or any other feeling that you do not normally experience. You may be sensitive to that medication, in which case the doctor will probably change the dosage or discontinue the drug. NOTE: Alcohol is a drug, and other drugs may not mix well with it, especially oral hypoglyacemic agents. See ALLERGY.

DRUGS, STORAGE OF *Keep all medication out of the reach of children.* Ideally, all medications are kept in a cool, dry place. Container caps should be secured tightly. Always keep the medicine in the original container; fancy pillboxes may not keep them fresh, or safe from children. Leave desiccants in containers. All drugs should have an expiration date on the container; do not use after the date of expiration. Clean out the medicine cabinet regularly and destroy all old medicines by flushing them down the toilet.

The daily insulin dose should come from a bottle kept at average room temperature, around 70°F (21°C). If the room gets very hot, over 90°F (32°C), or goes to freezing temperatures at night, it is best to store the insulin in the refrigerator. The butter-storage compartment is an ideal location. Be sure to remove the insulin an hour before using. Keep extra insulin supplies in the refrigerator, but do not allow them to freeze. For storage of reagent strips and tablets for urine

71

testing, see URINE TESTS.

DRY SKIN   See SKIN CARE.

DUCTLESS GLANDS   See GLANDS

DULCITOL   See Sugar Substitutes under SUGAR.

DUODENAL ULCER   See ULCERS.

DUPUYTREN'S CONTRACTURE   A progressive contracture of the hand in which the fingers, especially the third and fourth fingers, are pulled in toward the palm of the hand. It is painless, affects mostly males, has a high incidence with increasing age, and is observed in diabetics more than in the general population. Surgery has been employed to improve severe contracture.

DYE   See RADIOPAQUE DYE.

DYSCRASIA   See BLOOD DYSCRASIA.

DYSENTERY   See DIARRHOEA.

DYSFUNCTION   Inability or difficulty in the functioning of an organ or system.

DYSPHAGIA   Difficulty in swallowing.

DYSPNOEA   Difficulty in breathing. See also AIR HUNGER; ALLERGY.

DYSURIA   Painful or difficult urination that is most often due to infection (cystitis). See also URINE TESTS.

E

EARLY-ONSET DIABETES   See Diabetes Mellitus, Juvenile-Onset under DIABETES MELLITUS.

EAR NOISES   See TINNITUS.

EATING BETWEEN MEALS   See Use of Snacks under FOOD EXCHANGES.

EATING OUT   See TRAVELLING WITH DIABETES.

ECG   See ELECTROCARDIOGRAM.

ECLAMPSIA   See PREGNANCY AND CHILDBIRTH; TOXAEMIA OF PREGNANCY.

EGGS   See FOOD EXCHANGES, List 5.

EKG   See ELECTROCARDIOGRAM.

ELECTROCARDIOGRAM (ECG or EKG)   A recording made by an electrocardiograph picturing the electrical forces made by the heart as it beats. It is a painless test that takes only a few minutes. From the ECG the doctor can diagnose abnormal heart rhythms, heart enlargement, and some types of heart disease. An exercise, or stress, ECG is an ECG taken while the patient is performing his daily work and exercise, or on a treadmill in the doctor's surgery or laboratory. See also HEART DISEASE.

ELECTROPHORESIS   A laboratory test to separate and identify substances by their size and electrical charge. It is used in the tests for triglycerides, for cholesterol when the various densities of lipoproteins are desired, and in other tests for blood proteins such as albumin and globulins. See also BLOOD TESTS; LIPIDS.

ELECTROLYTES   All body fluids contain chemical compounds or substances classed as electrolytes or non-electrolytes. Electrolytes are those compounds that when in solution are capable of conducting an electric current; they are thus able to carry material from one place to another. Electrolytes break up or dissociate in water into ions (Greek – 'wanderers'), which are either positively or negatively charged. Positive charges, called cations, are attracted to negative poles, or cathodes; negative charges, called anions, are attracted to the positive poles, or anodes.

The major electrolytes in the human body are the cations sodium (Na+) and potassium (K+), and the anions chloride (C1−) and bicarbonate (HCO₃−). These ions are largely responsible for movement of the body fluids between tissues, maintenance of the acid-base balance and control of body water volume.

Electrolytes are lost mainly through the kidneys, but smaller amounts are also lost through the lungs, bowels, and skin.

Abnormal and often critical electrolyte loss occurs with dehydration, high fever, heatstroke, vomiting, diarrhoea, diabetic ketoacidosis, lactic acidosis, and the alkalosis of hyperglycaemic hyperosmolar nonketotic coma. See also ACID-BASE BALANCE, BLOOD TESTS; OSMOSIS, OSMOTIC DIURESIS.

ELECTROMYOGRAM (EMG) To test the action of a muscle, an electrical stimulus is applied and the response is recorded.

ELECTRORETINOGRAM See RETINA, RETINOPATHY.

EMBRYO The earliest stage of development of an organism. In humans it is a term applied to the period from the fertilisation of the ovum until all organs and major structures have been formed, usually 7 to 9 weeks. After this time, the developing baby is called a foetus. See PREGNANCY AND CHILDBIRTH.

EMERGENCIES See APPENDIX D; EMERGENCIES.

EMESIS See VOMITING

EMG See ELECTROMYOGRAM.

EMOTIONS These can change as the level of blood glucose changes, especially when it goes down. Becoming irritable or unreasonable may be the sole sign of low blood glucose. Listen to your family or friends – they may be the first to know. Emotional changes also make diabetes harder to control. See also Living with Diabetes under DIABETES MELLITUS; HYPOGLYCAEMIC REACTIONS.

EMPLOYMENT Most diabetics have better-than-average work records, with 70 per cent or more companies employing diabetics. Be honest with your employer about having diabetes. Your doctor can give the company the information it needs about your health; some large companies do routine laboratory tests for their diabetic employees. A diabetic can perform heavy manual labour, or be a professional athlete, but there are some jobs a diabetic should avoid, especially if he takes insulin – for example, flying, driving a public vehicle, or working on a scaffold. Write to the British Diabetic Association* for job information.

EMULSIFY To disperse minute gobules or particles of one liquid throughout another.

ENDOCRINE GLANDS OR SYSTEM See GLANDS.

ENDOCRINOLOGIST An internist who specialises in the treatment of diseases of the endocrine system. See also INTERNIST; DIABETOLOGIST.

ENDOGENOUS Made within body cells. Endogenous insulin is insulin made by the beta cells of the pancreas.

ENERGY NEEDS FOR SPECIAL ACTIVITIES See EXERCISE/SPORTS (includes a diet for exercise).

ENTEROPATHY Nerve damage to the alimentary canal. See DIABETIC NEUROPATHY.

ENURESIS Loss of urine by accident, such as bedwetting; it is called 'urinary incontinence' as a general term, and 'nocturia' when it happens at night. Damage to the nerves serving the urinary bladder is one cause of incontinence. See also DIABETIC NEUROPATHY.

ENZYMES All cells contain protein catalysts called enzymes, which accelerate the speed of cellular reactions. Every reaction that takes place within the cell requires a specific enzyme.

In general, enzymes are named by addinbetic neuropathy.

ENURESIS Loss of urine by accident, such as bedwetting; it is called 'urinary incontinence' as a general term, and 'nocturia' when it happens at night. Damage to the nerves serving the urinary bladder ee also BLOOD; BLOOD TESTS.

EPIDEMIOLOGY The study of how often a disease occurs and how it spreads.

*See Directory

EPIDERMIS   The outer layer of the skin.

EPISTAXIS   See NOSEBLEED.

ERUCTATION   Belching. See INDIGESTION.

ERYTHEMA   Redness of the skin. See also ALLERGY; ITCHING; SKIN CARE.

ERYTHROCYTES   Red blood cells. See also BLOOD.

ESSENTIAL AMINO ACIDS (EAA)   See AMINO ACIDS.

ESSENTIAL FATTY ACIDS   See LIPIDS.

ESSENTIAL HYPERTENSION   See BLOOD PRESSURE.

ETHNIC DIETS   See discussion of ethnic diets and Exchange Lists for Ethnic Foods under FOOD EXCHANGES.

ETHYL ALCOHOL (Ethanol)   The drinking type of alcohol. See ALCOHOL.

EUGLOCON   See ORAL HYPOGLYCAEMIC AGENTS.

EVAPORATED MILK   See FOOD EXCHANGES, List 1, Milk Exchanges.

EXACERBATION   The return of symptoms, or the worsening of a sickness.

EXCHANGE DIETS   See FOOD EXCHANGES.

EXCHANGE DIET SYSTEM   See FOOD EXCHANGES.

EXCHANGE LISTS   See FOOD EXCHANGES.

EXCORIATION   Abrasion of the skin or any organ of the body. It can be caused by chemicals, injury, burns and rubbing; also by urine and sweat. See BED SORES; SKIN CARE.

EXCRETION   The process of ridding the body of waste, including stool and urine, or the loss of water and salts by sweating. The lungs are also a major excretory organ.

EXERCISE DIET   See EXERCISE/SPORTS.

EXERCISE ECG   See ELECTROCARDIOGRAM.

EXERCISE/SPORTS   At one time it was thought that exercise was bad for the diabetic, but it is now known that exercise is one of the best things a diabetic can do to increase the effectiveness of insulin. Many famous athletes were or are diabetics. For a while it was not known why insulin works better in an active body; now it is felt that when energy needs are greater than dietary intake, as in exercise (when you are exercising you aren't eating), free fatty acids and ketone bodies are made available to muscle and fat tissue in a complex glucagon/insulin/glucose relationship.

Basic Rules in Sports and Exercise
1. Don't work-out alone!
2. Try to be as consistent as possible and exercise the same amount every day. When you engage in extra exercise, such as weekend skiing, take along dextrose cubes (available at most sport-shops), Dextrosol, or other favourite quick-acting sugars. Be sure your companions know you have diabetes and are aware of the symptoms of and treatment for a hypoglycaemic reaction.
3. Discuss food-habits, exercise, and insulin dosages at length with your doctor. When you do this, it will help you both if you take along careful records showing food intake, insulin dosage, urine tests, and the time and severity of any hypoglycaemic reactions you may have had. Some doctors are adamant that the insulin dose should not be changed, and athletes as a group seem to feel that they have better control if they eat more food, rather than decreasing the insulin dose. It is important that you remember to eat regularly – come in off the slope or take along a lunch. Being a good sport does not mean being foolish.

Swimming   This is the best sport of all because it uses so many muscles and can be undertaken at many levels and at any age. Strenuous swimming uses extra calories, and so does cold water. *Do not swim alone!* Take swimming lessons; learn water-safety. If you are used to swimming in a pool, remember that lake and ocean swimming are different – don't take on too much. Water may be cold; currents may be strong. Be aware that the sandy bottoms at ocean beaches, even in the same spot, tend to change with the wind and tides from day to day, sometimes even from hour to hour.

Diet for Exercise   A probable bonus to exercise and sports is weight loss and improved use of insulin – your own insulin, or injected insulin. The following is a Diet for Added Physical Activity† for diabetics:

Physical activity determines the rate at which energy is

†Reprinted from the Kaiser-Permanente Diet Manual, Southern California Region, with the permission of Mary E. Wilson, RD, former clinical dietitian, Permanente Medical Group Clinic, Fontana, California.

utilsed. Good diabetic control requires a regular programme of activity. Not only is the amount of activity important, but its consistency as well. Any important change in physical activity requires adjustments in the diabetic programme. This is especially vital for the insulin dependent diabetic.

It is difficult to give the exact amount of food required for various activities because this will vary from one person to another depending on how quickly they use energy, and how fast they walk, run, swim, etc. You will need to adjust your intake of food according to your own personal needs.

Below is given a very rough estimate of the amount of energy required for several common activities. The energy used is for an 11 stone individual. These figures are to be used only as a guide in helping you to determine the amount of food you need for various physical activities.

PHYSICAL ACTIVITIES	CALORIES USED PER MINUTE	EXTRA CALORIES USED PER MINUTE OVER EXPENDITURE FOR RECLINING
Reclining	1.3	
Walking*	5.2	3.9
Bike Riding**	8.2	6.9
Swimming***	11.2	9.9

*Walking 3.5 miles per hour on level ground (this is fairly brisk walking).
**Riding on level ground.
***Energy required for actual swimming; no extra food is required for sitting at poolside!

KAISER-PERMANENTE TABLE OF DIET FOR EXERCISE

The amounts of foods recommended are to be eaten *in addition to* your normal daily meal plan; they are based on the difference between the number of calories required for reclining (which has already been planned in your diet) and the number of calories required per minute for each activity.

ACTIVITY TIME	ENERGY USED (Cals)	AMOUNT OF FOOD TO HAVE BEFORE ACTIVITY	SAMPLE MENU	AMOUNT OF FOOD TO HAVE AFTER ACTIVITY	SAMPLE MENU
		WALKING			
½ hr	117	1 Milk Exchange	1 cup skim milk	1 Fruit Exchange	1 small apple
1 hr	234	½ Milk Exchange	½ cup skim milk	1 Fruit Exchange	1 small apple
		1 Bread Exchange	1 slice bread		
		1 Meat Exchange	1 oz roast beef		
		BICYCLE RIDING			
½ hr	207	1 Milk Exchange	1 cup skim milk	1 Fruit Exchange	1 small apple
		1 Bread Exchange	2 (2½″ sq.) graham crackers		
1 hr	414	1 Milk Exchange	1 cup skim milk	1 Fruit Exchange	1 small apple
		2 Bread Exchanges	2 slices bread		
		1 Meat Exchange	1 oz roast beef		

(Table continued on next page)

ACTIVITY TIME	ENERGY USED (Cals)	AMOUNT OF FOOD TO HAVE BEFORE ACTIVITY	SAMPLE MENU	AMOUNT OF FOOD TO HAVE AFTER ACTIVITY	SAMPLE MENU
		BICYCLE RIDING (cont.)			
1 hr		2 Fat Exchanges	2 tsp mayonnaise		
		SWIMMING			
½ hr	297	1 Milk Exchange	1 cup skim milk	1 Fruit Exchange	1 small apple
		1 Bread Exchange	1 slice bread		
		1 Meat Exchange	1 oz roast beef		
		1 Fat Exchange	1 tsp mayonnaise		
1 hr	594	1 Milk Exchange	1 cup skim milk	1 Fruit Exchange	½ cup orange juice
		2 Bread Exchanges	2 slices bread	1 Bread Exchange	4 strips melba toast
		2 Meat Exchanges	2 oz roast beef	1 Meat Exchange	¼ cup cottage cheese
		1 Fat Exchange	1 tsp mayonnaise		

EXPANDED LIST OF ENERGY REQUIREMENTS
FOR SPECIAL ACTIVITIES†

ACTIVITY	CALORIES/ HOUR
Bicycling 5 mph	264
Bicycling 9.5 mph	420
Bicycling 13 mph	659
Bowling	222
Carpentry	228
Climbing stairs	609
Dancing – ballroom	367
Dancing – square	441
Driving auto	147
Driving truck	294
Fishing	222
Gardening	367
Golf (no cart)	294
Golf (cart)	222
Handball	882
Hiking	441
Horseback riding	257
Housework	180*
Hunting	441
Labour – heavy	810
Labour – manual	420
Lawn mowing – hand-push mower	270*
Lawn mowing – power mower	250*
Mecanical work on car	183
Playing cards	147
Roller skating	350
Running 5.5 mph	609
Running 8 mph	1,008
Sewing	99
Sitting	84

†Adapted from *The Lazy Man's Guide to Physical Fitness,* Kenneth D. Rose, MD, with Jack Dies Martin, Greatlakes Living Press, Matteson, Illinois, 1974.
*Taken from other sources.

ACTIVITY	CALORIES/ HOUR
Skiing – downhill	588
Skiing – cross-country	1,197
Sleeping	67
Standing – relaxed	93
Sweeping floors	172
Swimming ¼ mph	300
Swimming backstroke 40 yds/min	609
Swimming crawl 50 yds/min	798
Table tennis	294
Tennis	588
Typing	103
Walking 2 mph	189
Walking 3 mph	264
Walking 4 mph	336
Water skiing	441
Writing	99

EXOGENOUS Originating from outside the body. Exogenous insulin is insulin injected into the body or infused into the veins.

EXPIRATION DATE See DRUGS, STORAGE OF.

EXTENDED INSULIN ZINC SUSPENSION Ultralente Insulin. See INSULIN.

EXUDATES Materials that have escaped from blood vessels. See also EYESIGHT.

'EYEBALL' To eyeball food is a slang expression meaning to judge the right quantities of food just by looking at it. It is better at first to weigh or measure foodstuffs, and periodically check your 'eyeball' measurement. This is especially true if you experience a weight gain or a positive urine glucose test.

EYESIGHT If you have trouble with vision – for example, blurring that occurs abruptly – it may be an indication that blood sugar is too low (hypoglycaemia). However, if the problem develops gradually, check for sugar and acetone in the urine, take your temperature, and call the doctor; you may have acidosis. Poor eyesight that has been developing over a period of time – weeks, months, or even years – may be a sign that diabetes control is not good. Double vision (diplopia), blurred vision, or dancing lights are all suspicious signs of glaucoma, and should be check by a doctor. See also RETINA, RETINOPATHY.

Some eye problems can be handled with a change in diet, and some require surgery and other techniques. Perhaps your glasses need changing. Be sure to keep appointments with your eye doctor and ask to see him more often if problems arise.

Lens The lens of the eye is the transparent structure just beneath the pupil through which light is gathered and projected into the nerve centre or retina at the back of the eye. See also RETINA, RETINOPATHY for diseases of the retina. See also BLINDNESS; ULTRASONOGRAPHY.

Cataracts A clouding of the lens of the eye. When levels of glucose are high in poorly controlled diabetes, and there is too little insulin, glucose may take alternate pathways called polyol or sorbitol pathways. Polyols, which are sugar alcohols (see SUGAR), collect in the lens and can cause cataracts. The traditional surgery for cataracts is the removal of the lens intact. Phaco-emulsification is a new technique in which the surgeon makes a very small opening and, using an ultrasound instrument, breaks up and sucks out pieces of the lens. After cataract surgery, intraocular lenses made of plastic may be put in place of the natural lens. This plastic lens is usually fitted for seeing at a distance. Regular eyeglasses must be used to see close up.

Audio and Visual Aids Most libraries lend large-print books and magazines. For details of special services for the blind and visually handicapped, contact the RNIB*.

Several special syringes are available for the visually handicapped. See INSULIN SYRINGES AND THEIR CARE.

EYETONE REFLECTANCE COLORIMETER See Dextrostix under BLOOD TESTS; RESEARCH.

*See Directory.

F

FAD DIETS See DIET; WEIGHT.

FAECAL IMPACTION See CONSTIPATION.

FAHRENHEIT (F) A unit of temperature measurement. The normal body temperature is around 98.6 F. For conversion to Celsius, see METRIC SYSTEM. See also THERMO-METER, CLINICAL.

FALSE-POSITIVE TEST A test that tests as positive but may not actually be positive because of a variety of interfering factors. See URINE TESTS.

FALSE TEETH See MOUTH CARE.

FAMILIAL Referring to traits or diseases that tend to occur in families. Diabetes runs in families to some degree. See also HEREDITY.

FAMILIES OF DIABETICS See Living with Diabetes under DIABETES MELLITUS.

FAMILY PLANNING ASSOCIATION A non-profit making organisation which gives advice on matters relating to birth control, infertility and sexual difficulties.

FAST-FOOD RESTAURANTS See FOOD EXCHANGES.

FASTING To go without eating. Some tests require fasting for some hours before the test. Chief among these are the tests for triglycerides (12 to 14 hours or overnight), and most tests measuring glucose in the blood. Instructions are generally given by the doctor or nurse. If water is not mentioned, ask; many tests require water so that urine may be produced as part of the test. Most testing procedures allow water but not tea or coffee, even if they are taken plain.

Fasting to achieve weight loss is an extreme measure and should never be undertaken without medical supervision. Starving the body slows the use of glucose, releasing fat stores and resulting in the use of fatty acids as food. In starvation an acetest will be read positive as in ketosis. See also BLOOD TESTS; KETONE BODIES.

FASTING BLOOD SUGAR (FBS) Also called 'fasting blood

glucose'. See BLOOD TESTS.

FAT BABIES The idea that a fat baby is a healthy baby is not necessarily true. According to Dr Leo P. Krall of Harvard University and the Joslin Clinic in Boston, a fat baby has an 85 per cent chance of becoming a fat adult. In addition, if a baby weighs over 9 or 10 pounds at birth the mother's chance of developing diabetes increases in later life if she does not already have it. See DIABETOGENIC; PREGNANCY AND CHILDBIRTH.

FAT DETERMINATION STOOL COLLECTION A laboratory test to determine the amount of fat in the stool (faeces) and to help in the diagnosis of disease. For three days before taking the test, follow a normal diet or a diet as ordered by your doctor. The doctor may also request a sample of stool weighing at least 5 grams (about 1 teaspoon), collected in a stool-specimen cup, which he will give you; or he may order a three-day sample. This should be collected from a bedpan and saved in a special container from the laboratory. Too much fat in the stool is called steatorrhoea. It may be caused by poorly controlled insulin-dependent diabetes, inflammation of the pancreas, or pancreatic cancer, as well as many other less sinister conditions.

FAT EXCHANGES OR CHOICES See FOOD EXCHANGES, List 6.

FATIGUE Being tired can be a sign of low blood glucose or poor health in general. See also HYPOGLYCAEMIC REACTIONS; LACTIC ACID.

FATNESS See WEIGHT.

FATS AND FATLIKE SUBSTANCES All fats, animal, vegetable, solid or oils, yield 9 calories/gram as food. In the past, diabetic diets were designed to supply about 40 per cent of the daily calories in fat; however, today many doctors are using much less fat in diet prescriptions – some as low as 15 to 20 per cent. Fats that are used as food and energy can be changed and stored as glucose, but they are stored mostly as fat. Insulin is not required to use fat as food, so in the absence of other food or insulin or both, fat is used as food with the breakdown into fatty acids and acetone. See also GLUCOSE POTENTIAL OF FOODS; KETONE BODIES; LIPIDS; URINE TESTS.

FATTY ACIDS See LIPIDS.

FBS Fasting Blood Sugar. See BLOOD TESTS.

FEBRILE See FEVER.

FED STATE Opposite of fasting. In the fed state, insulin secretion is stimulated and glucagon is decreased.

FEELING-LOSS See ANAESTHESIA.

FEET, CARE OF In the diabetic, loss of feeling and poor blood circulation are fairly common. This means the diabetic foot is more likely to become irritated or otherwise injured and is more open to infection. Athlete's foot (dermatophytosis), caused by a fungus, can infect the foot that is insensitive to pain; even more serious, gangrene, which may be caused by a bacterium *(Clostridium perfringens)* found in soil, can infect an unnoticed or unheeded cut.

For general foot care, wash and inspect the feet carefully every day. Wash them in warm (not hot) water with a mild soap. Take care of blisters, cracks, cuts, athlete's foot, corns, calluses, or splinters at once. It is a good idea to discuss foot care with the doctor. Apply skin lotion if you like. Do not put cotton between the toes, because the fibres can irritate; use gauze instead. Do not use pumice stone on the feet – pieces of stone can get into the skin, create a sore, and invite infection. You may soak your feet, but *do not* use hot water – a temperature below 110°F (43.4°C) is safe. *Do not* use Epsom salts. If you need a foot soak, see a doctor and take his advice.

Wear clean socks or hose. Cotton or wool or a combination is best. Women can wear ordinary hose so long as they cause no special problems, but they must fit well, with room for toe movement and with no wrinkles to irritate the skin. Do not wear tight girdles, garters, or elastics to hold up hose.

Shoes must also fit well. Wear new shoes only for short periods until they are comfortable. Do not wear the same pair two days in a row.

And, of course, *never go barefoot!* Rubber thongs are poor substitutes for shoes, because they give little protection to the toes and the soles may be easily punctured.

At night, turn on the lights when you get up and keep a night-light on in dark areas of the home. Always keep a torch by the bed and in the car to minimise the danger of stubbing your toes and bruising your shins.

Toenails   Toenails must be cut straight across, taking extreme care to avoid cutting the skin. The best time to cut the nails is after a bath or shower. White spots on nails may be evidence of a fungus infection. Thick, cracked, or deformed toenails should be cared for by a chiropodist.

Bunions   The joints of the big toes can become swollen, tender, and infected. Diabetics should be especially careful of bunions; see a chiropodist for treatment.

Hammer-toes are common in diabetics, and shoes should be fitted to provide adequate room to prevent irritation in this area.

Well-fitting shoes do not produce corns; however, if you have a corn *do not* cut it yourself. Ask a chiropodist to take care of it.

Foot pain   Foot pain without apparent injury may accompany leg pain or may occur alone. The type of pain varies from a dull ache or cramp to severe lightning-like pain, sometimes worse at night. It is often relieved by getting up and walking about. The pain may be due to blood vessel or nervous system disease; improved diabetic control may improve or completely relieve the condition. See also DIABETIC NEUROPATHY; LEG PAIN.

FERMENTATION TEST FOR SUGAR   See URINE TESTS.

FEVER   A rise in the body temperature above the normal. Sweating may accompany a high fever, with the result that the body may lose a lot of water, increasing the fever. When fever is present, be sure to drink plenty of fluids. Report temperature and results of urine testing for glucose and acetone to the doctor. See THERMOMETER, CLINICAL.

FIBRE   Also called roughage. More fibre in the diet may help lower blood glucose levels in some patients; however, do not put yourself on a high-fibre diet without first consulting your doctor.

High-fibre diets may also help relieve constipation, because fibre absorbs water when eaten and makes softer, larger stools. Fibre is found in seeds, fruits, roots, stems, flowers, and leaves of plants. Foods high in fibre are rolled oats, whole wheat, brown rice, buckwheat groats, leafy green vegetables, artichokes, celery, broccoli, Brussels sprouts, cabbage, cauliflower, and lettuce. Carrots, radishes, turnips, yams, beans, peas, corn, unpeeled potatoes, green peppers, pumpkin, okra, parsnips, apples, pears, peaches, blueberries, blackberries, and nuts are also good sources of fibre. See also CONSTIPATION; LAXATIVES.

FINGERNAILS See HANDS.

FINGERSTICK Sticking or piercing the fingertip to use with Dextrostix for blood glucose determination. The earlobe is also used as a stick-site. See also BLOOD TESTS.

FIRST-VOIDED URINE SPECIMEN See URINE TESTS

FISH See FOOD EXCHANGES, List 5.

FIVE-DROP CLINITEST See URINE TESTS.

FLOUR See FOOD EXCHANGES, List 4.

FLU See INFLUENZA.

FLUIDS Fluids can be given by a tube inserted by way of the nose or mouth directly into the stomach (nasogastric or NG tube); by rectum, by vein (IV); or by long needles directly into the tissues (hypodermoclysis). Fluids are normally lost through urine, stools, sweat, and lungs. See also DEHYDRATION; DIET; INTAKE AND OUTPUT.

FLUSHING A feeling of facial warming that can be caused by the vitamin niacin (nicotinic acid), menopausal changes, or using alcohol with oral hypoglycaemic agents.

FOETUS The term for an unborn baby from the end of about the seventh week of pregnancy up to birth.

FOLEY CATHETER See CATHETER.

FOLIC ACID (Folacin) A vitamin in the B group. It is found in leafy green vegetables, liver, meats, and fish.

FOOD ADDITIVES Substances added to food to enhance flavour or prevent spoilage. Salt, sugar, and spices are examples. Be sure to read the labels on food packages and containers to detect added sugar, and do not be fooled by fancy names for sugar, such as corn syrup, corn sweeteners, dextrose, sucrose, or lactose. If you are on a low-salt diet, check for salt or other sodium compounds. See also FOOD FLAVOURINGS; SODIUM; SUGAR.

FOOD EXCHANGES A food exchange can be a serving, allowance, choice, or portion. The exchange lists given here are taken from *Exchange Lists for Meal Planning,* prepared jointly by the American Diabetes Association and the American Dietetic Association. This booklet was updated in 1976 to reflect the current thinking by nutritionists that caloric intake and fat intake should be lower than was formerly recommended. A system of **boldface** type is used in the booklet and in this book to indicate those foods that contain low fat and/or polyunsaturate fat (see LIPIDS).

The basic food exchanges are divided into six groups, or lists. All the items in a given group have the equivalent caloric value. For example, an item on the fruit list, a scant ½ cup of orange juice, has the same number of calories as 1 cup of strawberries, 10 large cherries, or ½ slice of watermelon (10″ × ¾″). An exchange can be made only within a group – a fat for a fat, a fruit for a fruit, or a lean meat for a lean meat. A fat cannot be exchanged for a meat or for a fruit, even though it may have the same number of calories.

The lists offer a variety of food to eat, probably a greater variety than many people realise. For additional foods, consult the *Diabetic Diet Guide* available from the Joslin Diabetes Foundation. See also APPENDIX B: COOKBOOKS; FOODS TO AVOID; FREE FOODS.

For a 1,500-calorie sample diet, see page 100. For Use of Snacks, see page 101. For Vegetarian Food Exchanges, see page 102. For Fast-Food Restaurant Exchanges, see page 103.

FOOD EXCHANGES**

LIST 1. Milk Exchanges (includes **nonfat**, low-fat, and whole milk). *One Exchange of Milk contains 12 grams of carbohydrate, 8 grams of protein, a trace of fat, and 80 calories.*

There are good reasons for including milk as a basic food in your Meal Plan. It is the leading source of calcium. It is a good source of phosphorus, protein, some of the B-complex vitamins (including folic acid and vitamin B_{12}), and vitamins A

**Adapted from *Exchange Lists for Meal Planning;* used with permission of the American Diabetes Association and The American Dietetic Association.

and D. It also contains some magnesium.

Because milk is a basic ingredient in many recipes you will not find it difficult to include in your Meal Plan. Milk can be used not only to drink but can also be added to cereal, coffee, tea, and other foods.

The list shows the kinds and amounts of milk or milk products to use for one Milk Exchange. Those that appear in **bold type** are nonfat. Low-fat and whole milk contain saturated fat.

Nonfat fortified milk
Skim or nonfat milk	1 cup
Powdered (nonfat dry, before adding liquid)	⅓ cup
Canned, evaporated – skim milk	½ cup
Buttermilk made from skim milk	1 cup
Yoghurt made from skim milk (plain, unflavoured)	1 cup

Low-fat fortified milk
1% fat fortified milk	1 cup
(omit ½ Fat Exchange)	
2% fat fortified milk	1 cup
(omit 1 Fat Exchange)	
Yoghurt made from 2% fat fortified milk (plain, unflavoured)	1 cup
(omit 1 Fat Exchange)	

Whole milk (Omit 2 Fat Exchanges)
Whole milk	1 cup
Canned, evaporated whole milk	½ cup
Buttermilk made from whole milk	1 cup
Yoghurt made from whole milk (plain, unflavoured)	1 cup

LIST 2.   Vegetable Exchanges. *One Exchange of Vegetables contains about 5 grams of carbohydrate, 2 grams of protein and 25 calories.*

The generous use of many vegetables, served either alone or in other foods such as casseroles, soups or salads, contributes to sound health and vitality.

Dark-green and deep-yellow vegetables are among the

leading sources of vitamin A. Many vegetables in this group are notable sources of vitamin C – asparagus, broccoli, Brussels sprouts, cabbage, cauliflower, collards, kale, dandelion, mustard and turnip greens, spinach, rutabagas, tomatoes and turnips. A number, including broccoli, Brussels sprouts, greens, chard, and tomato juice, are particularly good sources of potassium. High folic acid values are found in asparagus, beetroot, broccoli, Brussels sprouts, cauliflower, collards, kale, and lettuce. Moderate amounts of vitamin B are supplied by broccoli, Brussels sprouts, cauliflower, collards, spinach, sauerkraut and tomatoes and tomato juice. Fibre is present in all vegetables.

Whether you serve them cooked or raw, wash all vegetables even though they look clean. If fat is added in the preparation, omit the equivalent number of Fat Exchanges. The average amount of fat contained in a Vegetable Exchange that is cooked with fat meat or other fats is one Fat Exchange.

This list shows the kinds of vegetables to use for one Vegetable Exchange. One Exchange is ½ cup.

Asparagus
Bean sprouts
Beetroot
Broccoli
Brussels sprouts
Cabbage
Carrots
Cauliflower
Celery
Courgettes
Cucumbers
Eggplant
Green pepper
Greens:
    Beetroot
    Chards
    Collards
    Dandelion

Greens
    Kale
    Mustard
    Spinach
    Turnip
Mushrooms
Okra
Onions
Rhubarb
Rutabaga
Sauerkraut
String beans, green or
    yellow
Tomatoes
Tomato juice
Turnips
Vegetable juice cocktail

The following **Raw Vegetables** may be used as desired:

Chicory	Lettuce
Chinese cabbage	Parsley
Endive	Radishes
Escarole	Watercress

Starchy Vegetables are found in the Bread Exchange List.

LIST 3.   Fruit Exchanges. *One Exchange of Fruit contains 10 grams of carbohydrate and 40 calories.*

Everyone likes to buy fresh fruits when they are at the height of their season. But you can also buy fresh fruits and freeze or can them for off-season use. For variety, serve fruit as a salad or in combination with other foods for dessert.

Fruits are valuable for vitamins, minerals, and fibre. Vitamin C is abundant in citrus fruits and fruit juices and is found in raspberries, strawberries, mangoes, cantaloupes, honeydews, and papayas. The better sources of vitamin A among these fruits include fresh or dried apricots, mangoes, cantaloupes, nectarines, yellow peaches, and persimmons. Oranges (and orange juice), and cantaloupe provide more folic acid than most of the other fruits in this listing. Many fruits are a valuable source of potassium, especially apricots, bananas, several of the berries, grapefruit, grapefruit juice, mangoes, cantaloupes, honeydews, nectarines, oranges (and orange juice), and peaches.

Fruit may be used fresh, dried, canned, or frozen, cooked or raw, as long as no sugar is added.

This list shows the kinds and amounts of fruits to use for one Fruit Exchange.

Apple	1 small
Apple cider	⅓ cup
Apple juice	⅓ cup
Applesauce (unsweetened)	½ cup
Apricots, fresh	2 medium
Apricots, dried	4 halves
Banana	½ small

Berries
    Blackberries   ½ cup
    Blueberries   ½ cup
    Raspberries   ½ cup
    Strawberries   ¾ cup
Cherries   10 large
Dates   2
Figs, fresh   1
Figs, dried   1
Grapefruit   ½
Grapefruit juice   ½ cup
Grapes   12
Grape juice   ¼ cup
Mango   ½ small
Melon
    Cantaloupe   ¼ small
    Honeydew   ⅛ medium
    Watermelon   1 cup
Nectarine   1 small
Orange   1 small
Orange juice   ½ cup
Papaya   ¾ cup
Peach   1 medium
Pear   1 small
Persimmon, native   1 medium
Pineapple   ½ cup
Pineapple juice   ⅓ cup
Plums   2 medium
Prunes   2 medium
Prune juice   ¼ cup
Raisins   2 tbsp
Tangerine   1 medium

Cranberries may be used as desired if no sugar is added.

LIST 4.   Bread Exchanges (includes **bread, cereal,** and **starchy vegetables**). *One Exchange of Bread contains 15 grams of carbohydrate, 2 grams of protein, and 70 calories.*

In this list, whole-grain and enriched breads and cereals, germ and bran products, and dried beans and peas are good sources of iron and among the better sources of thiamin. The whole-grain, bran and germ products have more fibre than products made from refined flours. Dried beans and peas are also good sources of fibre. Wheat germ, bran, fried beans, potatoes, parsnips, pumpkin, are particularly good sources of potassium. The better sources of folic acid in this listing include whole-wheat bread, wheat germ, dried beans, corn, parsnips, green peas, pumpkin, and sweet potatoes.

Starchy vegetables are included in this list because they contain the same amount of carbohydrate and protein as one slice of bread.

This list shows the kinds and amounts of breads, cereals, starchy vegetables, and prepared foods to use for Bread Exchange. Those that appear in **bold type** are low-fat.

Bread
White (including French and Italian)	1 slice
Whole wheat	1 slice
Rye or pumpernickel	1 slice
Raisin	1 slice
Bagel, small	½
English muffin, small	½
Plain roll, bread	1
Frankfurter roll	½
Hamburger bun	½
Dried bread crumbs	3 tbsp
Tortilla, 6″	1

Cereal
Bran flakes	½ cup
Other ready-to-eat unsweetened cereal	¾ cup
Puffed cereal (unfrosted)	1 cup
Cooked cereal	½ cup
Grits (cooked)	½ cup
Rice or barley (cooked)	½ cup

Pasta (cooked)
Spaghetti, noodles,
  macaroni   ½ cup
Popcorn (popped, no fat
  added)   3 cups
Cornmeal (dry)   2 tbsp
Flour   2½ tbsp
Wheat germ   ¼ cup
Crackers
Arrowroot   3
Mazoth, 4″ × 6″   ½
Oyster   20
Pretzels, 3⅛″ long × ⅛″ dia 25
Rye wafers, 2″ × 3½″   3
Soda, 2½″ sq   4
Dried beans, peas and lentils
Beans, peas, lentils
  (dried and cooked)   ½ cup
Baked beans, no pork
  (canned)   ¼ cup
Starchy vegetables
Corn   ⅓ cup
Corn on cob   1 small
Parsnips   ⅔ cup
Peas, green (canned or
  frozen)   ½ cup
Potato, white   1 small
Potato (mashed)   ½ cup
Pumpkin   ¾ cup
Winter squash, acorn or
  butternut   ½ cup
Yam or sweet potato   ¼ cup

Prepared Foods
  Biscuit, 2″ diam   1
    (omit 1 Fat Exchange)
  Corn bread, 2″ × 2″ × 1″   1
    (omit 1 Fat Exchange)
  Corn muffin, 2″ diam   1
    (omit 1 Fat Exchange)

Crackers, round butter type	5
(omit 1 Fat Exchange)	
Muffin, plain small	1
(omit 1 Fat Exchange)	
Potatoes, French fried, length	8
2" to 3½"	
(omit 1 Fat Exchange)	
Potato or corn chips	15
(omit 1 Fat Exchange)	
Pancake, 5" × ½"	1
(omit 1 Fat Exchange)	
Waffle, 5" × ½"	1
(omit 1 Fat Exchange)	

LIST 5.   Meat Exchanges. (A) Lean Meat. *One Exchange of Lean Meat (1 oz) contains 7 grams of protein, 3 grams of fat, and 55 calories.*

All the foods in the Meat Exchange lists are good sources of protein; many are also good sources of iron, zinc, vitamin B_{12} (present only in foods of animal origin), and other vitamins of the vitamin B complex. They are also sources of cholesterol, although lean meat contains less cholesterol than fat meat. (Foods of plant origin have no cholesterol.)

Oysters are outstanding for their high content of zinc. Crab, liver, trimmed lean meats, the dark muscle meat of turkey, dried beans and peas, and peanut butter all have much less zinc than oysters but are still good sources.

Dried beans, peas, and peanut butter are particularly good sources of magnesium and also of potassium.

Your choice of meat-groups throughout the week will depend on your blood lipid values. Consult with your dietician and your physician regarding your selection.

You may use the meat, fish, or other Meat Exchanges that are prepared for the family when no fat or flour has been added. If meat is fried, use the fat included in the Meal Plan. Meat juices with the fat removed may be used with meat or vegetables for added flavour. Be certain to trim off all visible fat, and measure meat after it has been cooked. A three-ounce serving of cooked meat is about equal to four ounces of raw meat.

To plan a diet low in saturated fat and cholesterol, choose only those Exchanges in **bold type**.

This list shows the kinds and amounts of **lean meat** and other protein-rich foods to use for one Low-Fat Meat Exchange.

Beef:	**chuck, flank steak, tenderloin, plate ribs, plate skirt steak, round (bottom, top), all cuts rump, spareribs, tripe**	**1oz**
Lamb:	**leg, rib, sirloin, loin (roast and chops), shank, shoulder**	**1 oz**
Pork:	**leg (whole rump, centre shank), ham, smoked (centre slices)**	**1 oz**
Veal:	**leg, loin, rib, shank, shoulder, cutlets**	**1 oz**
Poultry:	**meat without skin of chicken, turkey, pheasant**	**1 oz**
Fish:	**any fresh or frozen**	**1 oz**
	canned salmon, tuna, mackerel, crab, and lobster	**¼ cup**
	clams, oysters, scallops, shrimp	**5, or 1 oz**
	sardines, drained	**3 oz**
Cheeses containing less than 5 per cent butterfat		**1 oz**
Cottage cheese, dry and 2 per cent butterfat		**¼ cup**
Dried beans and peas (omit 1 Bread Exchange)		**½ cup**

(B) Medium-Fat Meat. *For each Exchange of Medium-Fat Meat omit ½ Fat Exchange.*

This list shows the kinds and amounts of medium-fat meat and other protein-rich foods to use for one Medium-Fat Meat Exchange.

Beef:	ground (15 per cent fat), corned beef (canned), rib eye, round (ground commercial)	1 oz
Pork:	loin (all cuts tenderloin), shoulder arm (picnic), shoulder blade, boiled ham	1 oz
Liver:	heart, kidney, and sweetbreads (these are high in cholesterol)	1 oz

Cottage cheese, creamed	¼ cup
Cheese: mozzarella, ricotta, farmer's cheese,	1 oz
Neufchâtel, Parmesan	3 tbsp
Eggs (high in cholesterol)	1
Peanut butter (omit 2 additional Fat Exchanges)	2 tbsp

(C) High-Fat Meat. *For each Exchange of High-Fat Meat omit 1 Fat Exchange.*

This list shows the kinds of high-fat meat and meat and other protein-rich foods to use for one High-Fat Meat Exchange.

Beef:	brisket, corned beef (brisket), ground beef (more than 20 per cent fat), hamburger (commercial), chuck (ground commercial), roasts (rib), steaks (club and rib	1 oz
Lamb:	breast	1 oz
Pork:	spareribs, loin (back ribs), pork (ground), country-style ham, devilled ham	1 oz
Veal:	breast	1 oz
Poultry:	capon, duck (domestic), goose	1 oz
Cheese:	cheddar types	1 oz
Cold cuts		4½" × ⅛" slice
Frankfurter		1 small

List 6.   Fat Exchanges. *One Exchange of Fat contains 5 grams of fat and 45 calories.*

Fats are of both animal and vegetable origin and range from liquid oils to hard fats.

Oils are fats that remain liquid at room temperature; they are usually of vegetable origin. Common fats obtained from vegetables are corn oil, olive oil, and peanut oil. Some of the common animal fats are butter and bacon fat.

Because all fats are concentrated sources of calories, foods on this list should be measured carefully to control weight. Margarine, butter, cream, and cream cheese contain vitamin

A. Use the fats on this list in the amounts shown on the Meal Plan.

This list shows the kinds and amounts of fat-containing foods to use for one Fat Exchange. To plan a diet low in saturated fat select only those Exchanges that appear in **bold type**. They are polyunsaturated.

Margarine, soft, tub or stick*	1 tsp
Avocado (4″ in diameter)**	⅛
Oil, corn, cottonseed, safflower, soy, sunflower	1 tsp
Oil, olive**	1 tsp
Oil peanut**	1 tsp
Olives**	5 small
Almonds**	10 whole
Pecans**	2 large whole
Peanuts**	
Spanish	20 whole
Virginia	10 whole
Walnuts	6 small
Nuts, other**	6 small
Margarine, regular stick	1 tsp
Butter	1 tsp
Bacon fat	1 tsp
Bacon, crisp	1 strip
Cream, light	2 tbsp
Cream, sour	2 tbsp
Cream, heavy	1 tbsp
Cream cheese	1 tbsp
French dressing***	1 tbsp
Italian dressing***	1 tbsp
Lard	1 tsp
Mayonnaise***	1 tsp
Salad dressing, mayonnaise type***	2 tsp
Salt pork	¾″ cube

*Made with corn, cottonseed, safflower, soy, or sunflower oil only.
**Fat content is primarily monounsaturated.
***If made with corn, cottonseed, safflower, soy, or sunflower oil, it can be used on a fat-modified diet.

SAMPLE 1500-CALORIE DIETS

1500 CALORIES (with milk)

Carbohydrate = 181 grams   Protein = 80 grams   Fat = 48 grams

BREAKFAST	NOON	EVENING
1 meat	2 meat	3 meat
1 bread	2 bread	2 bread
2 fruit	1 vegetable	1 vegetable
1 fat	2 fruit	2 fruit
1 low-fat milk	1 fat	1 fat
	1 low-fat milk	1 low-fat milk

1500 CALORIES (without milk)

Carbohydrate = 185 grams   Protein = 71 grams   Fat = 51 grams

BREAKFAST	NOON	EVENING
2 meat	2 meat	3 meat
3 bread	3 bread	3 bread
1 fruit	1 vegetable	1 vegetable
2 fat	1 fruit	2 fruit
	2 fat	2 fat

1500 CALORIES (with two snacks)**

BREAKFAST	NOON	EVENING
1 meat	2 meat	2 meat
1 bread	2 bread	2 bread
2 fruit	1 vegetable	1 vegetable
1 fat	2 fruit	1 fruit
1 low-fat milk	2 fat	1 fat
		1 low-fat milk

**See Use of Snacks.

100

Used with the permission of Charles H. Brinegar, Jr, MD, Assistant Professor of Medicine, Diabetologist, Loma Linda University School of Medicine, Loma Linda, California, and Margaret L. Kemmerer, RD, MS, Loma Linda University Medical Center,

USE OF SNACKS

Individuals with diabetes mellitus who are controlled by insulin or oral hypoglycaemic agents need appropriate spacing of carbohydrate, protein, and fat intake to help prevent hypoglycaemia. Afternoon and/or bedtime snacks may also be required to achieve stability of blood sugar levels.

Patients on three injections of soluble insulin per day, taken at the time of each meal, usually do not need snacks to stabilise their blood sugar between meals.

Intermediate-action insulin (NPH) reaches its peak effect 8 to 12 hours* after the injection, so it usually requires an afternoon snack to prevent hypoglycaemia.

Long-acting insulin taken by itself may not require an afternoon snack, but a substantial bedtime snack is recommended.

As a general safety precaution, a bedtime snack is suggested for all patients on insulin so that reactions do not occur during the night when they may not be aware of the symptoms. Often patients receiving one of the oral hypoglycaemic agents (sulphonylureas) should also have a bedtime snack.

Each snack should contain approximately 100 to 150 calories, including at least 5 grams of protein. The calories required for a snack are somewhat less for a very restricted calorie level, and larger snacks are given for very high calorie levels. The calories allowed for snacks should be part of the total calorie allotment for the day.

Suggestions for snacks that contain at least five grams of protein:

EXCHANGES	SAMPLES	CALORIES	GRAMS OF PROTEIN
1 meat choice	1 ounce cheese	55	7
½ bread choice	3 crackers	35	1
		90	8

*Latest figures indicate that intermediate-acting insulins (NPH) reach their peak of action in 6 to 8 hours.

EXCHANGES	SAMPLES	CALORIES	GRAMS OF PROTEIN
1 meat choice	¼ cup low-fat cottage cheese	55	7
1 fruit choice	½ cup DB* peaches	40	
		95	7
1 milk choice (nonfat)	1 cup nonfat milk	80	8
½ bread choice	1 cracker	35	1
		115	9
½ milk choice (nonfat)	½ cup nonfat milk	40	4
1 bread choice	1 slice bread + DB* jelly	70	2
		110	6
1 meat choice	1 slice cheese	55	7
½ milk choice (nonfat)	½ cup nonfat milk	40	4
		95	11
½ milk choice (nonfat)	½ cup nonfat milk	40	4
1 fruit choice	½ banana	40	
½ bread choice	3 crackers	35	1
		115	5

VEGETARIAN FOOD

MEAT-ALTERNATE EXCHANGE LISTS

Protein is found in various amounts in most plant foods. Two concentrated sources are wheat gluten and soybean fibre.

(continued on page 104)

*DB means 'diabetic', or without added sugar. In most cases, dietetic foods can be used, but be careful to check the nutritional labels. When in doubt, ask your doctor.

Food Exchanges for Fast-Food Restaurants

| | NUTRITIONAL VALUES | | | EXCHANGE VALUE | | |
	TOTAL CALORIES	CARBOHYDRATE (grams)	PROTEIN (grams)	FAT (grams)	BREAD	MEAT	FAT
Kentucky Fried Chicken (fried chicken, mashed potatoes, coleslaw, rolls)							
3-piece dinner							
Original	830	61	50	43	4	6	2½
Crispy	1070	74	54	62	5	6	6½
2-piece dinner							
Original	595	51	35	28	3½	2	1½
Crispy	665	40	37	40	3	4½	3½
McDonald's							
Hamburger	260	31	14	9	1½	1	1½
Double Hamburger	350	34	20	15	2	2	1
(make your own)							
Quarter pounder	420	37	25	19	2½	3	1
Big Mac	550	44	21	32	3	2	4
French Fries (chips)	180	20	3	10	1½	–	2
Chocolate Milk Shake	315	53	9	8	3½	–	1½
Pizza Hut (cheese pizza)							
Individual: thick crust	1030	143	71	19	9½	7½	–
thin crust	1005	128	61	28	8½	6	–
½ of 13" thick crust	900	113	65	21	7½	7	–
thin crust	850	103	50	26	7	5	–
½ of 15" thick crust	1200	148	83	31	10	9	–
thin crust	1150	144	66	35	9½	7	–

From 'Nutritional and Exchange Values for Foods' *Diabetes Forecast*, May–June, 1976. Used with permission of the American Diabetes Association.

Nuts also contain a liberal amount of protein. A variety of vegetable proteins can adequately replace flesh foods in a diabetic diet.

Vegetable protein meat alternatives are available canned or frozen; a few items are available in dehydrated form. A word of caution is in order here: Many of these products are supposedly 'ready to eat' but they taste their best when seasoned and prepared in combination with other ingredients. These items are completely heat processed as they are packaged.

PLANT PROTEIN FOOD*

The plant protein foods listed below contain carbohydrate and extra fat as well as protein. In most cases it is suggested that fruit instead of bread be omitted to compensate for this additional carbohydrate value.

BEANS AND PEAS	AMOUNT	EXCHANGE VALUE
Beans, all varieties (cooked)	½ cup (100 gm)	1 meat, 2 fruit; add ½ fat
Dried peas (cooked)	½ cup (100 gm)	1 meat, 2 fruit; add ½ fat
Lentils (cooked)	½ cup (100 gm)	1 meat, 2 fruit; add ½ fat
Soya beans, green (cooked)	⅓ cup (70 gm)	1 meat, ½ bread; add ⅓ fat
Soya bean curd (tofu)	½ cup (100 gm)	1 meat

NUTS AND SEEDS		
Peanuts	4 tbsp (30 gm)	1 meat, ½ fruit, and 2½ fat
Peanut butter	2 tbsp (30 gm)	1 meat, ½ fruit, and 2½ fat
Pistachio nuts	60 nuts (30 gm)	1 meat, ½ fruit, and 2½ fat
Walnuts	16–20 nuts (30 gm)	1 meat, ½ fruit, and 2½ fat
Cashew nuts	12–16 nuts (30 gm)	1 meat, ½ fruit, and 2½ fat
Sesame seeds	3 tbsp (30 gm)	1 meat, ½ fruit, and 2½ fat
Sunflower seeds	3 tbsp (30 gm)	1 meat, ½ fruit, and 2½ fat

*Used with the permission of Charles H. Brinegar, Jr, MD, Assistant Professor of Medicine, Diabetologist, Loma Linda University School of Medicine, Loma Linda, California, and Margaret L. Kemmerer, RD, MS, Loma Linda University Medical Center.

DIET SUPPLEMENTS

Wheat germ	3 tbsp (30 gm)	1 meat, 1 fruit
Yeast (brewer's)	3 tbsp (30 gm)	1 meat, 1 fruit; add 1 fat

Samples of 1,500-calorie vegetarian diets and snacks can be based on those already listed above, using meat substitutes.

For those whose diets and eating habits may vary according to their ethnic background, they may continue to follow those habits as long as their diets provide a nourishing variety of foods and stay within the bounds of the doctor's diet prescription.

Exchange Lists for Ethnic Foods

SPANISH FOOD	SERVING	EXCHANGE VALUE***
Ensalada de aquacite (sliced avocado with tomato and lettuce)		1 vegetable and 3 fats
Spanish omelet (eggs, peppers, tomatoes, onion)		2 meat and 1 fat
Chili verde (diced meat, green chili, rice or beans)		1 bread, 3 meat, and 2 fat
Corn tortilla	6-10" diam	1 bread
Flour tortilla	7-10" diam	1 bread and 1 fat
Taco shell	6" diam	1 bread and 1 fat
Chili con carne (no beans)	5 oz	1 meat and ½ bread
Chili con carne (with beans)		1 bread, 1 meat, and 1 fat
Tamale with sauce	1	1 meat and 1 bread
Spanish rice	1 cup	2 bread and 1 fat
Corn chips (taco and tortilla)	1 cup	1 bread and 2 fat
Chili sauce	2 tsp	1 fruit
Spanish sauce	½ cup	1 fruit and 1 fat
Enchiladar (meat or cheese)	6" tortilla	1 meat and 1 bread
Burrito, meat	10" flour tortilla	1 meat and 1 bread

***Exchange per average serving unless otherwise stated.

105

Burrito, beans	10" flour tortilla	2 breads
Chili relleno	7" long	2 meat and 1 bread
Taco (meat, cheese, tomato, lettuce)	7" tortilla	2 meat and 1 bread
Refried beans	½ cup	1 bread and 1 fat

ORIENTAL FOOD	SERVING	EXCHANGE VALUE
Ramaki (chicken livers, water chestnuts wrapped in beans)	2 pieces	1 meat and 1 fat
Shiu mi (chopped chestnuts, chives, and pork wrapped in thin noodle)	2 pieces	½ bread and ½ fat
Chow luny aas (fresh lobster tails in flavoured garlic sauce)	¾ cup	3 meat and 1 fat
Fung gawn aar (shrimp, chicken livers, mushrooms in chicken broth)	1 cup	3 meat and 2 fat
Mum yee mein (braised noodles, breast of chicken, mushrooms, chestnuts, Chinese peas)	1 cup	2 bread, 2 meat, and 1 fat
Seasonal vegetable and beef	1 cup	1½ meat and 1 vegetable
Egg flower sour	1 cup	½ meat
Fried rice (rice, meat, eggs, onions)	1 cup	1½ bread and ½ meat
Fortune cookie	2	1 bread
Egg roll	1	1 bread and 1 vegetable
Chow mein	1 cup	1 meat and ½ bread
Tofu	2 oz	½ meat
Sukiyaki	1 cup	3 meat and 1 fat
Chop suey	1 cup	2 meat and 1 vegetable
Pepper steak	1 cup	3 meat, 1 bread, and 1 vegetable
Chow mein noodles	½ cup	1 bread and 1 fat

ITALIAN FOOD	SERVING	EXCHANGE VALUE
Veal Parmigiana		4 meat, 1½ bread, and 1 fat
Italian spaghetti (with meatballs)		2 meat, 2 bread, and 1 fruit
Italian spaghetti (with tomato sauce)		2 bread and 1 fruit
Minestrone soup	½ cup	½ bread and 1 fat

Italian bread (with garlic butter)	1 slice	1 bread and 1 fat
Pizza (cheese, sausage, pepperoni)	$\frac{1}{6}$ (14-16 oz)	1 bread and $\frac{1}{2}$ meat
Ravioli (with beef)		1½ bread and 1 fat
Ravioli (with cheese)		1½ bread, ½ meat, and 1 fat
Lasagna		2 meat, 2 bread, 2 fat and 1 fruit

FOOD FLAVOURINGS (This category does not include food additives.) Herbs and spices of all kinds add pleasure to eating, and, unlike sugar, they have no calories. Some herbs and spices come in mixtures, which may cause trouble if the diabetic is on a low-salt (low-sodium) diet. Check all labels for salt content. You can add extra flavour to almost any dish: cheese sandwiches are tastier with a little dill-weed; omelettes with some chives, and tuna fish and tomato with a tiny bit of curry are surprising treats. One delicious use of mixed herbs is to sprinkle them lightly on fish and bake (poach) in a little milk. Alfalfa sprouts can be grown very easily by keeping the seed moist in a quart jar (special caps and seeds can be purchased in health food stores). It is fun to make up your own sandwich and salad recipes, and if they turn out well, to share them with others.

FOOD GROUPS See DIET.

FOOD POISONING A condition caused by eating food contaminated with bacteria, bacteria products (toxins), or poisonous foods such as certain types of mushroom. The symptoms are nausea, vomiting, abdominal pain, and diarrhoea. Contact your doctor immediately because an adjustment in your diabetic treatment will be needed for a few days.

FOOD PREPARATION See COOKING.

FOOD SUBSTITUTIONS See FOOD EXCHANGES.

FOODS TO AVOID Although most doctors permit a special diet for a special day such as a birthday party, the following list of foods should be avoided:

    1. Alcoholic drinks*
    2. Beer and ale (except diabetic lager)
    3. Wine*

*Some doctors will help you fit alcohol into your diet in small amounts.

4. Soft drinks with sugar
5. Condensed milk
6. Cookies
7. Cake
8. Doughnuts, sweet rolls
9. Candy
10. Pie
11. Gum, except sugarless
12. Honey
13. Jam and jelly
14. Marmalade
15. Preserves
16. Molasses
17. Sorghum
18. Sugars
19. Sugared cereals
20. Syrups

Almost all dietetic recipes, dietetic candy, and ice cream, and some coffee additives of the liquid kind should be avoided. Coffee-mate is limited to three or four teaspoons a day. See also DIET; DIETETIC FOOD; Sugar Substitutes under SUGAR.

FOOD VALUE The value of food in terms of energy available for use in the body has been measured in laboratories in terms of calories. In addition, food has been analysed to measure the amount of fat, carbohydrate, protein, vitamins, and minerals it contains. Other considerations in food value are its ease in digestion, the amount of fibre, and how storage and cooking affect its content. See also ALCOHOL; FOOD EXCHANGES; SUGAR.

FOOT CARE See FEET, CARE OF.

FOOT DROP Foot 'droop' is a more descriptive term. It can occur with nervous system disease (diabetic neuropathy), as a result of ineffective nerve stimulus to the muscles that flex the foot. With control of blood sugar, it usually gets better or disappears.

FOOT PAIN See FEET, CARE OF.

FORESKIN (Prepuce) See GENITALIA.

FORTIFIED NONFAT MILK See FOOD EXCHANGES, List 1.

FPA   The Family Planning Association.
FRACTIONAL URINE SPECIMEN   See URINE TESTS.
FREE DIET   See DIET.
FREE FATTY ACIDS (FFA)   See KETONE BODIES; LIPIDS.
FREE FOODS   These foods have little or no calories and may be included in the diet in any amounts:

Cereal beverages (such as Postum)	Pickles, sour*
Clear broth	Pickles, dill, unsweetened*
Coffee (black)	Noncaloric sweetening agents
Bouillon*	
Soft drink without sugar	Seasonings and herbs
Gelatine, unsweetened	Mustard*
Lemon	Vinegar
Rhubarb, sugarfree	Tabasco sauce
	Tea

   See also FOOD EXCHANGES; Sugar Substitutes under SUGAR.

FREEZING FOOD WITHOUT SUGAR   See CANNING AND FREEZING FOOD WITHOUT SUGAR.

FROZEN FOOD   Read the labels to make sure there is no sugar added to the food product (or salt if you are on a low-sodium diet). Use frozen foods the same way you use fresh or canned foods. Measure or weigh after cooking and draining, and save the cooking water for soup.

FRUCTOSE   See SUGAR.

FRUIT   See FOOD EXCHANGES, List 3.

FRUIT JUICE   Choose only unsweetened fruit juice and limit the intake as suggested by the doctor. Fruit juice used for a hypoglycaemic reaction should have no added sugar. See also FOOD EXCHANGES, List 3.

FRUIT SUGAR   Fructose (levulose). See SUGAR.

FRUITY BREATH   See ACETONE BREATH.

FULLY LIQUID DIET   See DIET.

FUNCTIONAL   Refers to how a system or part of a system works; for example, the function of the beta cells of the pancreas is to produce insulin, but this is a small part of the overall function of the endocrine system.

*Not for a low-sodium diet.

FUNCTIONAL REACTIVE HYPOGLYCAEMIA   See HYPO-
GLYCAEMIA.

FUNDASCOPE   See OPHTHALMOSCOPE.

FUNGUS   Yeasts and moulds. See MICRO-ORGANISMS.

FURUNCLE   A boil. See INFECTION AND INFLAMMA-
TION.

G

GALACTOSE See SUGAR.
GALL BLADDER See BILE; LIVER.
GALLONS See METRIC SYSTEM.
GAMES DIABETICS PLAY* We all tend to feel anxious in the face of the unknown. Some people attack a problem head on, accepting a situation, learning as much about it as they can, and making the required changes. Such adjustments are necessary for the diabetic to make in order to achieve control of his diabetes and his life. They have the additional benefit of allaying the feeling of helplessness that often accompanies the knowledge that one has the disease. But some diabetics do not manage this acceptance and adjustment. They will try to ignore the problem, or will use their diabetes as an excuse for avoiding living a normal life or as a means of manipulating others. Such people play a number of mental games to mask their anxiety and excuse their behaviour. The following are some typical statements made by diabetics as a way of avoiding reality:

1. I wish I did not have diabetes, so that I could hold down a steady job.
2. If I didn't have diabetes, I would be able to take trips and vacations.
3. I can't play tennis because of my diabetes.
4. I would like to remain on my diabetic diet, but I can't afford the expensive foods.
5. I know I should test my urine for sugar before lunch, but I can't do it because I am at school.
6. I don't understand how my blood sugar can be so high. Take a look at my urine tests for glucose. They are all negative.

*Adapted from 'The Care and Teaching of Diabetes', two-day seminar at Loma Linda University, November 1974. Used with permission of Jerome M. Feldman, MD, Director of Duke Diabetes Clinic, Duke University Medical Center, Durham, North Carolina.

7. I can't understand how I developed diabetic acidosis five times in a year. The only thing I did out of the ordinary was to have some cake for dessert Tuesday night.
8. I don't understand why I am so overweight. I do not eat any more food than my nondiabetic friends.
9. I know I should lose weight and stop smoking cigarettes, but I just cannot eliminate these bad habits.
10. Why should I develop diabetes? I never did anything to deserve such a fate.

GANGRENE See FEET, CARE OF.

GASTRIC Refers to the stomach.

GASTRITIS Inflammation of the stomach. It can happen in diabetic ketoacidosis.

GASTROINTESTINAL TRACT (GI Tract) Refers to the stomach and intestines together. If nerve damage is present, diabetics may have GI problems such as difficulty in swallowing (dysphagia), a slow emptying of the stomach, and either a delayed or rapid emptying of the intestines (constipation or diarrhoea). See also CONSTIPATION; DIABETIC NEUROPATHY; DIARRHOEA.

GENERAL PRACTITIONER (GP) A physician who does not limit his practice to one medical speciality.

GENERIC As applied to drugs, the official name of a drug or medicine under which it is listed by the pharmacopoea. For example, the generic name for the oral hypoglacaemic agent Orinase is tolbutamide; Orinase is a trade name used for promotional purposes by the Upjohn Company.

Although there are some exceptions, a drug manufactured and sold under the generic name is of the same quality as one sold under a trade name.

GENES; GENE LOCUS See CELLS.

GENETIC COUNSELLING See HEREDITY.

GENETIC ENGINEERING See RESEARCH (Recombinant DNA).

GENITALIA The sex organs, or organs of reproduction. In the male the internal organs consist of several glands and passageways or ducts for secretions, including sperm. The exposed parts are the penis and the testicles. In the uncircumcised male, the end of the penis is protected by the foreskin, or prepuce, which must be pulled back so that the penis may be cleaned thoroughly at least once a day. The foreskin should then be replaced. The urinary meatus, through which the bladder is emptied and seminal fluid expelled, is at the end of the penis.

In the female, the internal organs are the ovaries, the Fallopian tubes, the uterus, and the vagina. The external parts, the vulva, include the labia (lips), clitoris, urinary meatus and glands for the secretion of a lubricating fluid to aid in sexual intercourse.

Both male and female genitalia can become infected with micro-organisms, especially by a yeast called *Candida albicans*. Keep the genitalia clean and report any discharge, itching, burning, or sores to your doctor, because infection can make diabetes harder to control. Females should apply toilet paper in a front-to-rear direction to avoid infecting the urinary meatus and the vagina with bacteria from faeces. See also CANDIDA ALBICANS; URINARY BLADDER.

GENITOURINARY TRACT (GU Tract)   Refers to the urinary tract and genitalia together.

GERIATRICS   The medical treatment of the elderly.

GERMAN MEASLES   See MEASLES.

GERONTOLOGY   The study of the problems of ageing.

GESTATION   See PREGNANCY AND CHILDBIRTH.

GESTATIONAL DIABETES   See PREGNANCY AND CHILDBIRTH.

GI TRACT   See GASTROINTESTINAL TRACT.

GIN   See ALCOHOL.

GINGIVITIS   See MOUTH CARE.

GLAND   A cell, organ, or tissue that manufactures and secretes a substance that is used in another part of the body. There are three types of glands: endocrine, exocrine, and mixed endocrine-exocrine. The main endocrine glands are the thyroid and parathyroids, adrenals, pituitary, testes, ovaries, and the alpha, beta, and delta cells of the pancreas. Endocrine glands are ductless; that is, the secretions enter the blood stream and from there go to the body cells. Insulin is an example of an endocrine secretion. Exocrine glands secrete directly to tissue without entering the bloodstream;

113

some of them have ducts or passageways to an organ, and some secrete directly to an organ. Exocrine secretions serving the skin and linings of organs are secreted directly to those tissues. See also ADRENAL GLANDS; PANCREAS; PITUITARY GLAND; THYMUS GLAND; THYROID GLAND.

GLASS SYRINGES See INSULIN SYRINGES AND THEIR CARE.

GLAUCOMA See EYESIGHT; RETINA, RETINOPATHY.

GLIBENCLAMIDE Daonil or Euclogon. See ORAL HYPO-GLYCAEMIC AGENTS.

GLIPIZIDE Glibenese. See ORAL HYPOGLYCAEMIC AGENTS.

GLOBIN ZINC INSULIN (Globin Insulin) See INSULIN.

GLOBULINS A protein substance in the blood. For immuno-globulins, see ALLERGY.

GLOMERULUS See KIDNEYS.

GLOVE AND STOCKING EFFECT See PARAESTHESIA.

GLUCAGON A protein hormone secreted by the alpha cells of the pancreas. The main function of glucagon is to raise the blood glucose level. Similarly, in the nondiabetic the presence of glucose decreases the secretion of glucagon (and increases secretion of insulin). However, this effect is lost or lessened in the diabetic. In diabetic ketoacidosis some patients may have very high levels of glucagon; this produces high levels of glucose in the fasting state by stimulating the liver to produce glucose. High levels of glucagon have also been found in hyperglycaemic hyperosmolar nonketotic coma (HHNK), pancreatitis, obesity, liver cirrhosis, burns, infection, and surgery.

When carbohydrate is eaten, a bi-normal response takes place, which results in more insulin and less glucagon, suggesting that diabetes is a two-hormone disease; however, recent research suggests that a high glucagon level does not lead to onset of diabetes as long as the body is able to secrete enough insulin. The development of diabetes is probably more closely related to lack of insulin than to excess glucagon. This area is one of controversy at this time.

Injecting glucagon as an emergency treatment for severe hypoglycaemic reaction includes three important considerations: when to give it; how to give it; and what to do after giving it. This should be discussed with your doctor. Usually, glucagon is injected when sugar and other quick-acting carbohydrates cannot be given, that is, when the person is unconscious or otherwise unable to swallow. The drug, available only by prescription, is packed in a small kit containing two vials and instructions for use. One vial contains a powder and the other a diluent, or liquid, to mix with the powder. To mix, wipe the tops of both vials with an alcohol swab; withdraw the diluent by means of a syringe, and inject it into the vial containing the powder. This mixture makes 1 mg (or 1 cc) of glucagon. The usual procedure is to mix it when needed, but the mixture will keep three months in the refrigerator. (Mark the date mixed on the vial.) A 1 cc insulin syringe can be used. Glucagon can be injected subcutaneously like insulin, or intramuscularly with a longer needle if you know how to do it. Never give an injection into the buttock of a baby or very small child unless you are experienced; the muscle usually used in the child is the thigh muscle called the vastus lateralis found about halfway between the knee and the point where the thigh attaches to the body. Draw an imaginary line down the centre of the thigh, and inject at a point one-finger's width toward the outside of the thigh on a baby or small child, and two-fingers' width on a larger person. It is safe to use the gluteus maximus, a large muscle in the upper, outer fourth of the buttock in the large child or adult. Ask the doctor or nurse to locate these safe spots for injection. Draw a picture of these spots and place the drawing in the kit. An injection in the wrong place can mean serious and permanent nerve damage. Recommended doses are 0.5 to 1 mg (½ to 1 cc), or according to the doctor's order. If the person involved is a baby or a very small child, be sure to ask the doctor how much to give. The patient should awaken in 5 to 20 minutes. The doctor, meanwhile, should be notified, and he may ask to see the patient or have him taken to the nearest hospital. The effect of glucagon lasts for about an hour, and the patient will need sugar or glucose to build up his glycogen stores. Long-acting carbohydrates will also be given as soon as the patient is able to eat.

GLUCAGONOMAS　See TUMOURS.

GLUCAGON TEST　See BLOOD TESTS; GLUCAGON.

GLUCOCHEK　A portable electronic device for reading the colour of a Dextrostix strip. Manufactured by Medistron. (See Directory).

GLUCOCORTICOIDS　Hormones produced by the adrenal cortex. In response to inflammation or infection, they elevate blood glucose levels by increasing the manufacture of glucose from sources other than carbohydrate, (see GLUCONEOGENESIS), and blocking or antagonising the effect of insulin. Elevated blood glucose helps fight infection by supplying the metabolic requirements of the cells, which increase in the presence of infection. See ADRENAL GLANDS.

GLUCONEOGENESIS　In the liver, this is the process of making glucose from sources other than carbohydrate, that is, from protein and fat. See LIVER.

GLUCOSE　This is the sugar commonly meant when the term 'blood sugar' is used; it is the sugar measured in blood and urine tests. Glucose is a single sugar (a monosaccharide) and is the most important source of energy in the body. The brain and some other tissues use glucose exclusively, although ketone bodies can be utilised by the brain in the absence of glucose for a limited period of time.

In the past, blood glucose levels were indicated most often by using percentages present in whole blood. However, most of today's testing equipment is designed to measure values using plasma or serum, which do not ne tests. Glucose is a single sugar (a monosaccharide) and is the most important source of energy in the body. The brain and some other tissues use glucose exclusively, although ketone bodies can be utilised by the brain in the absenctage of glucose present in the blood. Serum and plasma glucose levels are normally 15 to 20 per cent higher than whole blood levels. Normal fasting values of glucose in plasma or serum are 80 to 120 mg/dl; in whole blood they are 60 to 100 mg/dl. In most British laboratories, different units are employed, the normal fasting blood glucose being 3.5 to 6 mmol per litre.

The abbreviation 'dl' stands for decilitre, $\frac{1}{10}$ of a litre, or

100 ml or cc. Older ways of expressing the same value are mg per cent (%), or mg per 100 ml or cc (mg/100ml). All mean the same thing. See also BLOOD TEST; METRIC SYSTEM; SUGAR; URINE TESTS.

GLUCOSE DRINK   See Oral Glucose Tolerance Test under BLOOD TESTS.

GLUCOSE EXCRETION   See Twenty-four-Hour Urine Collection under URINE TESTS.

GLUCOSE PASTE   See INSTANT GLUCOSE.

GLUCOSE POTENTIAL OF FOODS   Glucose can be made by the body from protein and fats as well as from carbohydrates. The diagram below shows the percentages of glucose that can be produced by these three foods.

Glucose is the number one source of energy for all cells, and must be in the blood in an amount necessary to support life. If the amount of glucose is less than 50 mg/dl, then the brain can suffer serious damage. (This is an average figure and there are exceptions.)

GLUCOSE POTENTIAL OF FOODS

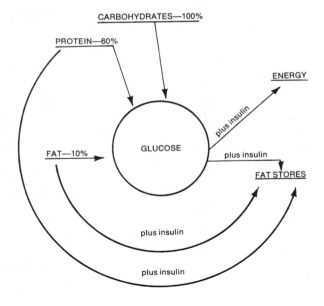

117

When the energy needs are met, the liver and muscle cells can change glucose into glycogen for storage. Glucose can also be converted into fat for storage. Some amino acids (glucogenic amino acids) can also be converted into glucose or glycogen.

GLUCOSE TOLERANCE/INTOLERANCE   The average person has a tolerance for sugar, because he has enough insulin to process it in the body. This is not to say sugar is good for the body. It is not. It causes tooth decay and stresses insulin supplies and other mechanisms having to do with glucose metabolism. The prediabetic and the diabetic, however, do not have enough effective insulin and are glucose intolerant.

Glucose tolerance is decreased by sickness or other physical and mental stress. It also decreases with age.

There are different degrees of glucose intolerance, but generally speaking, anyone with glucose intolerance is diabetic, or may become so with increasing years, obesity, lack of exercise, and improper diet.

GLUCOSE TOLERANCE TEST (GTT)   See Oral Glucose Tolerance Test under BLOOD TESTS.

GLUCOSE TOLERANCE TEST – INTRAVENOUS (IV)   See BLOOD TESTS.

GLUCOSURIA   See GLYCOSURIA.

GLYCAEMIA   Glucose in the blood. See HYPERGLY-CAEMIA.

GLYCEROL   See LIPIDS.

GLYCOGEN   A polysaccharide, or starch, known as animal starch. It is the form in which glucose is stored in the liver and muscles; it is converted to glucose and used as energy whenever glucose is unavailable. See also GLYCO-GENOLYSIS.

GLYCOGENESIS   When the blood glucose level is too high (hyperglycaemia), the liver attempts to lower it to normal by coverting glucose to glycogen. See also LIVER.

GLYCOGENOLYSIS   The conversion of glycogen to glucose. When the blood sugar is low, stored glycogen is split and released as glucose. See also LIVER.

GLYCOLIPIDS   A combination of carbohydrates and lipids. See also LIPIDS.

GLYCOLYSIS The release of energy from glucose. See also KREBS CYCLE.

GLYCOSURIA Glucose in the urine. Normal urine has 0.01 per cent glucose, although on rare occasions sugars other than glucose may be detected in the urine. See also MELI-TURIA; RENAL THRESHOLD; URINE TESTS.

GLYMIDINE Gondafon. See ORAL HYPOGLYCAEMIC AGENTS.

GOAT'S MILK Contains about the same number of calories as whole cow's milk and can replace it. See also FOOD EXCHANGES, List 1.

GONDAFON See ORAL HYPOGLYCAEMIC AGENTS.

GRAIN (gr) See METRIC SYSTEM.

GRAINS See FOOD EXCHANGES, List 4.

GRAM (Gm, gm, or g) See METRIC SYSTEM.

GRANULES; GRANULOCYTES See BLOOD.

GRIPPE See INFLUENZA.

GROWTH HORMONE Secreted from the pituitary gland, growth hormone, together with insulin, promotes body growth (protein synthesis). At the same time it raises blood glucose levels and is listed as an insulin antagonist. The latter effect is so slow, however, that it is secondary to the promotion of protein synthesis.

GROWTH-ONSET DIABETES See DIABETES MELLITUS, JUVENILE-ONSET.

GULLET See OESOPHAGUS.

GUM One stick of chewing gum (3 grams) has 10 calories and 2.9 grams of sugar. It is not good for your teeth. If you chew gum, use artifically sweetened gum. See also SUGAR.

GUMS See MOUTH CARE.

GUT See INTESTINES.

GU TRACT See GENITOURINARY TRACT.

H

HAEMATOCRIT (Packed Cell Volume) See BLOOD TESTS.

HAEMATURIA Blood in the urine. May be present in chronic kidney disease or in urinary tract infections.

HAEMOCHROMATOSIS (Bronze Diabetes) A liver disease caused by excess iron in the body. It occurs mostly in males. It is called 'bronze' diabetes because 90 per cent of the patients have a grey, dark tan, or bronze colour to the skin. Also called 'pigmentary cirrhosis'. There is involvement of the pancreas and 75 to 80 per cent of the patients may develop diabetes mellitus.

HAEMODIALYSIS See Dialysis under KIDNEY DISEASE.

HAEMOGLOBIN See BLOOD; BLOOD TESTS.

HAEMOGLOBIN A$_1$ See page 209.

HAEMORRHAGE See BLEEDING; RETINA, RETINO-PATHY.

HAEMORRHOIDS See VARICOSE VEINS.

HANDS Be careful of cuts, splinters, burns, allergies, blisters – any of these can become infected. Dishwater can be hot enough to burn the skin, especially if there is loss of feeling. Use mild soap and wear rubber gloves. Wear gloves when gardening, and let someone else prune the roses. Be careful when trimming fingernails not to cut the skin. See INFECTION AND INFLAMMATION; SKIN CARE.

HARDENING OF THE ARTERIES Arteriosclerosis. See HEART DISEASE.

HEADACHES Everyone occasionally suffers from headaches, so if a diabetic has a headache it may not be related to his diabetes. Headaches, however, may occur with a drop in blood glucose. As with all individuals, diabetics differ, making it impossible to say when this kind of headache may develop, how severe it might be, or how long it will last. If you suspect low blood glucose is the cause of the headache, drink a half cup of orange juice, and if the headache is relieved, low blood glucose was probably the cause. A urine test for glucose at this time may be positive because of previously elevated blood glucose levels, but a second-voided specimen would be negative. If this type of headache is a common occurrence, be sure to add this information to your records to help the doctor adjust your food intake or insulin schedule.

Migraine Headache   A severely painful headache, accompanied by nausea, stomach pains, and so on, which is caused by spasms of blood vessels and occurs on one side of the head only (unilateral). It is a recurring condition but, for reasons not understood, may disappear when diabetes is diagnosed and controlled.

Tension Headache   A headache caused by stress, which can often be relieved by massaging the head from the forehead, down the sides, over the ears, and down the neck on either side of the spinal column. Tight muscles, which can cause these headaches, are felt as little hard knots and are sore to the touch. Firmness combined with gentleness is the key to the massage. The knots will massage away, and usually all or much of the pain will go with them. If the headache returns, repeat the massage. See STRESS.

HEALTH INSURANCE   See INSURANCE.

HEARING LOSS   See NERVE DEAFNESS.

HEART ATTACK   See HEART DISEASE.

HEARTBEAT   See PALPITATION.

HEARTBURN   See INDIGESTION.

HEART DISEASE   Over half a million people in the United States die each year from coronary heart disease when the coronary arteries feeding the heart become occluded (clogged) and can no longer deliver blood to the heart muscle (myocardium). One half of these deaths are said to be related to diabetes as macroangiopathy (see BLOOD VESSEL DISEASE). Another half a million people survive heart attacks with prompt and skilful medical management.

Occlusion of coronary arteries is caused by the presence of fatty-fibrous lesion called plaques, or atheromas. The disease process is called atherosclerosis, and can be present in arteries throughout the body. Partially occluded arteries may be completely shut off by clots breaking away from

121

lesions and travelling in the arteries until they reach a place too narrow for them to pass. This event is called coronary thrombosis. It is thought that heredity, obesity, a diet high in saturated fats (see LIPIDS), excessive intake of sugar, and perhaps of alcohol, lack of exercise, and cigarette smoking are primary factors in atherosclerotic heart disease. An older word, arteriosclerosis, is a more general term referring to the disease of larger arteries that results in the stenosis or narrowing of blood vessels. See Circulation of the Blood under BLOOD.

The lives of those lucky half-million who survive a heart attack can be managed in various ways. There is today a popular technique called coronary bypass surgery. In this procedure a section of the clogged coronary artery is surgically removed and a vein from the patient's leg grafted in its place. The surgery is expensive and traumatic, and current research indicates that these substitute arteries usually become clogged in a few years. The alternative to bypass surgery is a medical regimen or treatment that is meeting with some success in the reversal of atherosclerosis. Featured in this programme is weight reduction, a diet that is low in saturated fat, and that emphasises polyunsaturated fats, cessation of smoking, and an exercise programme under the careful direction of a physician. Besides a new lease on life, a bonus to this treatment is a new sense of well-being, and for the diabetic, better control of his diabetes. See LIPIDS.

Everyone is concerned about the pain of heart disease. Angina pectoris means 'pain in the chest muscles'. Different people describe this pain in different ways; they may report that it feels like indigestion, or that it is crushing, as though the chest were in a vice. Typically, the pain originates in the oxygen-starved heart muscle, spreads across the chest to the left arm or to both arms, and may even be felt in the jaws, teeth, and forehead. An angina attack rarely lasts less than 30 seconds, or longer than 30 minutes. The medical treatment consists of nitrates, which dilate the blood vessels and allow blood to get through. Nitroglycerin (NTG) is the drug most often used; it is placed under the tongue (sublingually) and allowed to dissolve. If one or two tablets do not relieve the pain in 5 to 10 minutes, this may indicate an acute attack, which can result in damage to the heart muscle. This is called a myocardial infarction. 'Infarct' refers to an area of the heart tissue that is damaged and dies. (The word for dead tissue is necrosis.) This is always serious. In this case the pain tends to be a feeling of great pressure, occurring on the midline of the body; midchest, or anywhere from the upper abdomen to the neck. The patient will often feel short of breath, perspire, and feel great anxiety. Immediate hospitalisation is imperative!

A silent heart attack is one in which there is some damage to the myocardium, with little or no pain to warn the victim, and a spontaneous recovery. An electrocardiogram will probably show some heart damage; therefore, it is important to see your doctor at least once a year with follow-up visits as he may suggest.

Congestive heart failure (CHF) is caused by a heart that fails to perform adequately. Fluids collect in the lungs (congestion) or in the entire circulatory system or both. CHF is due to many causes, but whatever the cause, there is extra stress on the body, which complicates the control of diabetes, not only in fluid management, but because stress and inactivity may make blood glucose levels harder to control.

Tests to determine the degree of heart disease are of great importance in the treatment. These tests include the measurement of various enzymes, lipids in the blood, angiography, and ultrasonography (see all).

HEATING PADS   See BURNS.

HEIGHT TABLES   See WEIGHT.

HEPATIC   See HAEMOCHROMATOSIS.

HEPATITIS   Inflammation of the liver. Viruses are among the causes of hepatitis, particularly the infectious and serum hepatitis viruses.

HEPATOMEGALY   Enlargement of the liver. See LIVER DISEASE.

HERBS   See CONDIMENTS; FOOD FLAVOURINGS.

HEREDITY   Diabetes mellitus is inheritable to some degree.
The following tables list the prediction of diabetic risk.

ADULT-ONSET DIABETES*

PRIMARY RELATIVE WITH DIABETES MELLITUS		OTHER DIABETIC RELATIVES	MAXIMUM RISK
Parent	plus	Grandparent *plus* aunt or uncle	85%
Parent	plus	Grandparent *or* aunt or uncle	60%
Parent	plus	First cousin	40%
Parent			22%
Grandparent			14%
First cousin			9%

JUVENILE-ONSET DIABETES**

ONE PARENT DIABETIC	BOTH PARENTS DIABETIC	ONE SIBLING DIABETIC	MORE THAN ONE SIBLING DIABETIC	ABSOLUTE RISK FOR CHILD†
+	−	−	−	5%
−	+	−	−	10–15%
+	−	+	−	10%
−	+	+	−	20%
−	−	+	−	5%
−	−	−	+	10%

The facts are that at this time no one really is sure how diabetes is passed on from one generation to another, especially in the juvenile type. There seems to be a more positive genetic factor in juvenile-onset diabetes than in adult-onset diabetes. Thus, genetic counselling is wise when diabetics marry, if only for peace of mind. The question of inheritance is far from settled, but a genetic counsellor can give you the facts as they are known, and let

---

*Based on figures published by P. White, P. Koshy, and J. Duckers. 'Management of pregnancy complicating diabetes and of children of diabetic mothers'. *M. Clin. Borth America* 37:1481. 1953.

**Adapted from material provided by Leo P. Krall, MD, Director, Education Division, Joslin Diabetes Foundation, Boston, Massachusetts. Used with permission.

†Approximate values.

the decision be your own as to whether you should have children. See also CELLS.

HHNK See HYPERGLYCAEMIC HYPEROSMOLAR NONKETOTIC COMA.

HIGH ALTITUDES See EXERCISE/SPORTS; TRAVELLING WITH DIABETES.

HIGH BLOOD PRESSURE See BLOOD PRESSURE.

HIGH BLOOD SUGAR See HYPERGLYCAEMIA.

HISTORICAL MILESTONES* Some of the important events in the history of diabetes mellitus are listed below:

DATE	EVENT	INVESTIGATORS
ca10	Clinical description	Celsus
ca20	Name diabetes introduced, meaning, in Greek, 'to run through'	Aretaeus
1679	Sweet taste of urine noted	Willis
1788	Pathology of pancreas in diabetes	Cawley
1850 et. seq.	Dietary restriction treatment – starvation	Bouchardat, von Noorden, Naunyn, Allen, E. P. Joslin, and others
1869	Discovery of pancreatic islets	Langerhans
1870	Sugar (glucose) storage in liver as glycogen and elevated blood sugar in diabetes	Bernard
1874	Overbreathing of diabetic acid poisoning	Kussmaul
1889	Experimental diabetes after pancreas removal (dog)	Von Mering and Minkowski
1895	Hereditary nature of diabetes; distinction between juvenile-onset and late-onset diabetes	Naunyn
1900	Islet lesions in diabetics	Opie, Weichselbaum and Stangle
1909	Hypothetical hormone of islets named 'insuline'	de Meyer

*Used with permission of Leo P. Krall, MD, Directory, Education Division, Joslin Diabetes Foundation, Boston, Massachusetts.

125

1910–1920	Insulin almost discovered	Zuelzer, Scott, Knowlton, and others
1913	Hypoglycaemia (low blood sugar) by oral guanidine, forerunner of DBI	Watanabe
1921	Insulin discovered (dog)	Banting and Best
1922	Insulin used in humans	Banting and Best
1923	Lessening of pancreatic diabetes by hypophysectomy (removal of pituitary)	Houssay
1936	PZI (Protamine Zinc Insulin)	Hagedorn (Denmark)
1936	Lessening of pancreatic diabetes by adrenalectomy in cat (removal of the adrenals)	Long, Lukens
1938	NPH insulin (Neutral Protamine Hagedorn)	Hagedorn (Denmark); Scott, Fisher (Canada)
1952	Lente insulin	Hallas-Moller (Denmark)
1955	Structure of insulin determined	Sanger
1955	'Pill' introduced – Carbutamide	Franke and Fuchs (Germany)
1956	Tolbutamide (Orinase)	Upjohn (United States)
1957	Phenethyl – biguanide (DBI)	US Vitamin (United States)
1958	Chlorpropamide (Diabinese)	Pfizer (United States)
1960	Immunoassay of insulin	Berson and Yalow
1963	Synthesis of insulin	Katsoyannis and Dixon
1964	Acetohexamide (Dymelor)	Lilly (United States)
1965	Tolazamide (Tolinase)	Upjohn (United States)
1968	Proinsulin	Steiner

Dr Elliot P. Joslin is responsible for naming the various eras for the men in which their work was outstanding:

Before 1914 – Naunyn   1936-1946 – Hagedorn
1914-1921 – Allen   1946 – Charles H. Best
1921-1936 – Banting

HOME CARE City or county health departments staffed with district nurses and health visitors make home visits to instruct in all phases of diabetic care as needed. Some departments have registered dietitians. This is a free service offered as a function of local government. Visiting nurses and private homecare organisations provide the same service in some areas, and are listed in the yellow pages of the telephone book under NURSES.

HOMEOSTASIS When all systems in the body are functioning properly, a state of balance exists called equilibrium or homeostasis. An example of imbalance is the acid-base imbalance of diabetic ketoacidosis. See also ACID-BASE BALANCE.

HONEY See SUGAR.

HONEYMOON PERIOD See REMISSION PERIOD.

HORMONES Chemical substances produced by glands that help regulate body functions. Insulin is a hormone. Premarin, an oestrogen birth-control pill can raise blood glucose. Be sure your doctor knows all the drugs you are taking even if they have been taken for a long time. See also CONTRACEPTIVES; DRUG PROFILE; PREGNANCY AND CHILDBIRTH.

HOT SOAKS See FEET, CARE OF; SKIN CARE.

HOT WATER BOTTLE See BURNS.

HUMAN MILK See PREGNANCY AND CHILDBIRTH.

HUNGER (at times other than mealtime) See HYPOGLYCAEMIC REACTIONS.

HYDRAMNIOS Same as Polyhydramnios. See PREGNANCY AND CHILDBIRTH; TOXAEMIA OF PREGNANCY.

HYDROGEN The simplest of all atoms, having only one electron.

HYDRATION Fluid replacement. See DEHYDRATION; FLUIDS.

HYDROGENATED FATS See LIPIDS.

HYDROLYSIS Any reaction with water.

HYPER- A prefix meaning above or more than normal; excessive.

HYPERCHOLESTEROLAEMIA See LIPIDS.

HYPERESTHAESIA See PARAESTHESIA.

HYPERGLUCAGONAEMIA Too much glucagon in the blood.

HYPERGLYCAEMIA A condition in which blood glucose is in excess of normal. Although the causes of hyperglycaemia

127

are many, the primary one is lack of effective insulin. The normal range of plasma glucose is generally accepted as between 3.5 and 6 mmol per litre, fasting.

The most common causes of hyperglycaemia are forgetting to take insulin, errors in dosage, infection, disease, stress, and improper diet containing concentrated carbohydrates (sugars). When the blood glucose levels exceed 10 mmol/L, glucose usually shows up in the urine. See also RENAL THRESHOLD; BLOOD TESTS; URINE TESTS.

HYPERGLYCAEMIC HYPEROSMOLAR NONKETOTIC COMA (HHNK) A very dangerous, newly recognised, metabolic problem caused by hyperglycaemia (high blood glucose) ranging from 40 to 100 mmol per litre and resulting in severe dehydration. As a complication of diabetes, it is most likely to be found in the undiagnosed diabetic, or in newly recognised cases.

There are many symptoms that relate to HHNK. In general, symptoms, in addition to high blood glucose and dehydration, are oliguria (lack of urine), low blood pressure, fever, visible signs of dehydration (including tenting of the skin and soft eyeballs; see DEHYDRATION), and confusion and disorientation progressing to lethargy, stupor, and coma if the condition is left unchecked.

Acidosis is not present, and there will therefore be no ketones in the urine. The patient with HHNK is very sick, and if not already hospitalised, will require immediate medical attention to lower the blood glucose and to replace fluids and the resulting electrolyte imbalances. See also ELECTROLYTES; OSMOSIS, OSMOTIC DIURESIS.

HYPERINSULINAEMIA Too much insulin in the blood.

HYPERINSULINISM Too much insulin produced by the pancreas. Many obese people and diabetics have more than the normal amount of insulin in the body, but are unable to use it because of the resistance of fat cells to insulin. Hyperinsulinism can also be caused by a tumour of the pancreas (insulinoma), or it can be caused by an oversensitivity of the beta cells in the pancreas in early diabetes to high blood glucose. See also TUMOURS.

HYPERLIPIDAEMIA An excess of lipids in the blood. See LIPIDS.

HYPERLIPOPROTEINAEMIA   See LIPIDS.

HYPERSENSITIVITY   A condition of more than normal sensitivity. See ALLERGY.

HYPEROSMOLAR COMA   See HYPERGLYCAEMIC HYPEROSMOLAR NONKETOTIC COMA.

HYPEROSMOLALITY   See OSMOSIS, OSMOTIC DIURESIS.

HYPERTENSION   See BLOOD PRESSURE.

HYPERTROPHY   An increase over normal in the size of an organ or a structure. For example, the liver can increase in size because of disease; a muscle can increase in size because of increased use; or, with insulin injection, bulges (hypertrophy) or indentations (atrophy) can occur when insulin is injected at one site too often. See also INSULIN INJECTION AND INJECTION SITES.

HYPERVENTILATION   Breathing faster than normal, more deeply than normal, or both. Usually caused by anxiety. Not the same as Kussmaul's respirations in diabetic ketoacidosis or lactic acidosis. See also AIR HUNGER.

HYPERVOLAEMIA   See CENTRAL NERVOUS PRESSURE.

HYPNOTIC   A drug that induces sleep. See NARCOTICS.

HYPO-   A prefix meaning below or less than normal.

HYPOCOUNT   A portable electronic device for reading the colour of a Dextrostix strip. Manufactured by Hypoguard. (See Directory.)

HYPODERMIC   Hypodermic means under the skin; the same as subcutaneous.

HYPOGLYCAEMIA   A less-than-normal amount of glucose in the blood. Hypoglycaemia has been called a 'nondisease', and many doctors feel that there is a tendency to overdiagnose the condition, but at the same time, they fully recognise that fact that some people have low blood glucose and that they have distressing symptoms caused by it. (See HYPOGLYCAEMIC REACTIONS.) Other people have low blood glucose with no symptoms or problems of any kind. Though hypoglycaemia is said to exist when the blood glucose is less than 2.5 mmol per litre, the Joslin Clinic in Boston found that 30 per cent of normal people (with no history of diabetes) have blood glucose levels of less than 2.5

mmol per litre; among prediabetics (those with a history of diabetes in the family, or with other criteria such as giving birth to large babies) only about 10 per cent drop to levels below 2.5 mmol per litre during an oral glucose tolerance test. Clearly, more studies must be done to determine what low blood glucose levels mean in the oral glucose tolerance test.

Hypoglycaemia is very common in persons who drink alcohol on an empty stomach. It is also caused iatrogenically; that is, by a doctor who prescribes too much insulin or too high a dose of oral hypoglycaemic agents, or by a patient who makes an error in the dose of either drug, fails to eat properly, or exercises too much without taking in extra food. See EXERCISE/SPORTS (includes a diet for exercise).

Paradoxically, when the blood glucose falls from a high level to a lower level at a fast rate – for example, from 30 mmol per litre to 10 mmol per litre, which is still high blood glucose state – a person may experience hypoglycaemic reactions, because the body cannot adjust that fast. This situation is usually caused by giving too large a dose of insulin in the treatment of high blood glucose. See HYPO-GLYCAEMIC REACTIONS; SLIDING-SCALE INSULIN COVERAGE.

Hypoglycaemic Coma A condition in which the blood glucose is so low that the brain does not receive enough glucose to function. This is to be avoided because of the danger of brain damage. See HYPOGLYCAEMIC REACTIONS.

Reactive Hypoglycaemia Sometimes called 'reactive functional hypoglycaemia', this is a condition in which the body responds to a physiological situation by a lowering of the blood glucose. Experts do not entirely agree on the definition of reactive hypoglycaemia, because so many of the symptoms are highly individual and sometimes bizarre; however, it seems safe to say that there are three general types.

    1. Emotionally induced: the blood glucose falls 2 to 4 hours after eating carbohydrates. See ADRENAL GLANDS.

2. Excessive insulin release: the blood glucose falls 3 to 5 hours after eating carbohydrates. This condition exists in many obese persons, and can be diagnostic in early or mild diabetes, but is now open to question.
3. After gastric surgery: the blood glucose falls ½ hour after eating carbohydrates because the stomach is unable to handle carbohydrates effectively. Also called the 'dumping syndrome'.

See Oral Glucose Tolerance Test under BLOOD TESTS.

HYPOGLYCAEMIC AGENTS Any drug or method used to reduce high blood glucose. Insulin and pills or capsules are used in conjunction with diet to lower the blood sugar. See also ORAL HYPOGLYCAEMIC AGENTS.

HYPOGLYCAEMIC COMA See HYPOGLYCAEMIA; HYPOGLYCAEMIC REACTIONS.

HYPOGLYCAEMIC REACTIONS When the blood glucose falls to a point low enough to effect a response in the nervous system, a group of symptoms collectively called 'hypoglycaemic reaction' or 'insulin reaction', may occur. The extreme forms of these reactions are also called 'insulin shock' and 'hypoglycaemic coma'.

A hypoglycaemic reaction is usually precipitated by the presence of too much insulin, either because an erroneous dose was given or because the patient has neglected to eat, or has failed to eat enough before strenuous exercise. Low blood glucose can also be caused by the excessive use of oral hypoglycaemic agents, although in this case the onset is usually slower and more insidious.

Whatever the cause, there are two important considerations of which the diabetic and his family and friends must be aware: (1) hypoglycaemic reactions must be avoided because of the danger of brain damage; and (2) the signs and symptoms, though varying with individuals, include nervousness or restlessness, shaking, hunger, pale skin, weakness and fatigue, headache, and sometimes sweating. The blood pressure may drop and the pulse rate may increase. These symptoms can be relieved by eating or drinking something sweet. It is best to discuss thoroughly with the doctor the possibility of a hypoglycaemic reaction before it occurs; if this has not been done, the most common action is to take about 10 grams of carbohydrate, which is one fruit exchange (see FOOD EXCHANGES, List 3). Quick home carbohydrates include ½ cup of orange juice (do not add sugar), ¼ cup of grape juice, ⅓ cup unsweetened apple juice or pineapple juice. Since it is not always convenient to carry juices, you can substitute for them ½ can of Coke or 7-Up (not the diet type), ½ candy bar, or 2 cubes of sugar. Not so handy, but effective, are 2 teaspoons of pancake syrup or honey. If you are working hard or exercising, *stop!* As soon as possible, eat some long-acting food such as ½ a sandwich, which will have to be subtracted from the next meal. Trial and error is the only way to judge what is best for you. Carry small cans of easy-to-open fruit juice in the car and dextrose sweets (Dextrosol) on your person at all times.

Early signs of low blood glucose may be entirely absent, or at least not apparent; however, changes in behaviour may be noticeable to those around. A diabetic can be fairly certain blood glucose is low if for no reason you feel impatient and irritated, or if you have difficulty concentrating.

Later signs of low blood glucose include sweating difficulty in seeing (having either blurred or double vision), dilated pupils, confusion, numbness, and stupor, which can lead to coma. Hypoglycaemic reactions may occur during sleep. Be suspicious if you have bad dreams or wake up very sweaty. Treatments of these later signs can be handled in the same way as early signs, so long as the person is fully able to swallow. Sweets should be repeated in 10 minutes if symptoms do not disappear. If the symptoms are so severe that the person's ability to swallow is impaired and danger from choking exists, Glucagon may be given. See GLUCAGON.

If the above treatments do not produce results in 20 minutes, the diabetic patient must be taken to the doctor or to the nearest hospital where intravenous 50 per cent glucose solution may be infused. The hospital staff should be made fully aware of what has been done for the patient at home.

Urine samples, if available, may be positive for glucose, especially on a first-voided specimen. This is because the urine in the bladder reflects the blood sugar level over a period of time and not at the moment. See also URINE TESTS.

If you are diabetic, be sure to *wear at all times an identification bracelet or necklace* that gives your name, address, nearest relative, doctor, phone numbers, and the information that you have diabetes. See MEDIC ALERT.

HYPOPHYSIS   See PITUITARY GLAND.

HYPOTENSION   See BLOOD PRESSURE.

HYPOTHALAMUS   A small structure in the brain near the pituitary gland that helps to control many functions in the body, including sugar and fat metabolism. Somatostatin, which inhibits growth hormone and glucagon secretion, is one of the products of the hypothalamus.

HYPOVENTILATION   Slow or shallow breath, or both. This is not the same as Kussmaul's respirations. See also AIR HUNGER.

HYPOVOLAEMIA   See CENTRAL VENOUS PRESSURE.

HYPOXIA   See AIR HUNGER; ANOXIA.

I

IAMAT International Association for Medical Assistance to Travellers. See TRAVELLING WITH DIABETES.

IATROGENIC *Iatro* is a Greek combining form that refers to a physician or to medicine. Iatrogenic means 'caused by a doctor'. An example of this would be when the doctor prescribes too large a dose of insulin, causing hypoglycaemia. Also, misunderstanding the doctor can cause worry and stress sufficient to affect the blood glucose, so always speak up if you have any doubts and ask him exactly what he means.

ICE BAG (Pack) Ice applied continuously can cause skin damage if left for periods over 15 minutes, especially if loss of feeling exists. Set an alarm clock in case you fall asleep.

ICE CREAM See IMITATION ICE CREAM, ICE MILK.

ICU See INTENSIVE CARE UNIT.

IDEAL BODY WEIGHT The amount you should weigh for your height, bone structure, sex, and age. See also WEIGHT.

IDENTICAL TWINS Twins that grow from a single egg, or ovum. In the past, it was believed that when one twin had diabetes, the other twin would also become diabetic. Recent research indicates that this is not true; of the adult-onset type, around 50 per cent may become diabetic, but of the juvenile-onset type, the figure is in dispute, but is thought by some to be considerably less than 50 per cent. See also HEREDITY.

IDENTIFICATION Always carry an identification card giving your name, address, nearest relative, doctor, phone numbers, and the information that you have diabetes. Include a list of medication being taken. Many drug companies and hospitals supply free cards for wallets. For bracelets and neck chains , see MEDIC ALERT.

IDF International Diabetes Foundation. See DIABETES ASSOCIATIONS.

IDIOPATHIC   A disease occurring without a known case.

IDIOPATHIC DIABETES MELLITUS   Diabetes in which the cause or reason is not known.

IDIOPATHIC INSULIN-RESISTANT DIABETES   See INSULIN-RESISTANT DIABETES.

ILETIN   Trade name of insulin manufactured by Eli Lilly Co. See INSULIN.

ILLNESS   See SICKNESS.

IM   See INTRAMUSCULAR INJECTION.

IMITATION ICE CREAM, ICE MILK   In imitation ice cream, the butterfat used in real ice cream is replaced by vegetable oil – usually coconut oil, which is highly saturated. In ice milk no fat is added. Both products contain sugar, making them unsuitable for the diabetic diet. Dietetic ice cream has sugar substitutes in place of sugar; however, it has other calories that must be figured into the total daily calories. See also DIETETIC FOOD; LIPIDS; Sugar Substitutes under SUGAR.

IMITATION MAYONNAISE   See MAYONNAISE.

IMMUNE REPONSE   See ALLERGY.

IMMUNOASSAY   A technical laboratory procedure used to measure the amount of certain substances in the body; for example, the amount of insulin present in the blood at a given time. Immunoassays utilise the reactions that occur when antigens are bound to antibodies. When radioactive materials are used, the term radioimmunoassay (RIA) is used. See ALLERGY.

IMMUNOGLOBULINS   See ALLERGY.

IMPACTION   See CONSTIPATION.

IMPOTENCE   The inability in the male to achieve an erection. Impotence that arises while the diabetes is poorly controlled often disappears when good control is established. Impotence can be caused by blood vessel disease, nervous system disease, or psychological reasons. Treatment is available either by your own doctor, or by a specialist he can recommend.

INACTIVITY   If you are inactive for whatever reason you may have to eat less, or increase the intake of insulin or oral hypoglycaemic agents. For reasons not fully understood, insulin is less effective during times of sickness or other periods when one is less active. Consult with the doctor if urine tests are positive for glucose and/or acetone.

INCONTINENCE See DIABETIC NEUROPATHY; ENURESIS.

INDIGESTION Incomplete or poor digestion that can cause stomach pain, nausea, vomiting, eructation (belching), diarrhoea, and heartburn. Heartburn tends to be in the upper gastric (stomach) area, especially in the oesophagus; a half-glass of skim milk often helps to relieve it. Indigestion can be accompanied by an elevation in body temperature (see THERMOMETER, CLINICAL); if so, report any fever along with urine test results for glucose and acetone to the doctor. See also SICKNESS.

INFANT OF THE DIABETIC MOTHER See PREGNANCY AND CHILDBIRTH.

INFARCTION See HEART DISEASE.

INFECTION AND INFLAMMATION The invasion of the body by pathogenic (disease-causing) micro-organisms. Infection can be as small as a pimple or as serious as a kidney or bladder infection. Most doctors believe that diabetics are more susceptible to infections than nondiabetics, especially if their diabetes is not well controlled, or if they do not take good care of their skin, feet, and genitalia.

Pus is a thick fluid that forms as a result of an infection. It can be smelly; thin or thick; practically colourless, yellow, reddish, or even greenish blue. It can occur anywhere in or on the body. Pus is composed of dead white blood cells (see BLOOD), dead bacteria, and tissue debris.

Inflammation may occur when tissue is injured or diseased; the body sends extra blood to the area for healing, and the increased volume of blood in the area can cause pain, heat, redness, and swelling. Infection may be present, causing a rise in body temperature. Follow the instructions under SICKNESS. See also BLOOD TESTS; CANDIDA ALBICANS; IMMUNE RESPONSE; MICRO-ORGANISMS; URINARY BLADDER.

INFLUENZA Also known as flu, or grippe, it is a virus infection with symptoms that usually occur abruptly and last four or five days. One feels sick, with symptoms that may include fever, aches and pains, sore throat, cough, nausea and vomiting, and diarrhoea. Antibiotics are not used in the treatment of influenza unless the influenza is complicated by a concurrent infection of a bacterium (see MICRO-ORGANISMS); in either case, however, flu is stressful to the body, and the diabetic will probably need help from the doctor.

INFUSION See INTRAVENOUS INFUSION.

INGROWN TOENAILS See FEET, CARE OF.

INHERITANCE OF DIABETES See HEREDITY.

INHIBITOR In the case of two or more drugs, an inhibitor is a drug that makes another work less efficiently, or have less effect than when used alone. Be sure your doctor knows about all the drugs you are taking. See also INSULIN ANTAGONIST; ORAL HYPOGLYCAEMIC AGENTS; POTENTIATION.

INJECTION SITES See INSULIN INJECTION AND INJECTION SITES.

INJURY See ACCIDENTS; INFECTION AND INFLAMMATION.

INOSITOL See Sugar Substitutes under SUGAR.

INSECTS See ALLERGY; BITES AND STINGS.

INSOMNIA The inability to sleep or, once asleep, to remain asleep. If insomnia makes the diabetes harder to control, ask your doctor for help, but do not take sleeping pills unless prescribed.

Instead of becoming restless or upset with tossing and turning, which can cause stress, try getting up, whatever time it is. Watch a late movie, read, write letters. Borrow a snack from your bedtime allotment or breakfast – milk, hot or cold, is often effective in bringing on sleep.

INSTANT NONFAT DRY MILK A packaged product. When water is added to the powder following the directions on the package, the mixture has the same food value as liquid nonfat milk. To make sure it taste as good as liquid milk, keep it refrigerated for 12 hours or more, but it can be used immediately in cooking. Skim milk contains more protein than whole milk on a percentage basis, and, of course, has no fat. See also FOOD EXCHANGES, List 1.

INSULIN A hormone secreted by the beta cells of the islets of Langerhans in the pancreas. It is the major building hormone in the body (See METABOLISM) and as such may be called the hormone of energy storage. Although exactly how insulin is released is not fully understood, it is felt that it is influenced by the digestive hormones of the upper intestine in response to the ingestion of food, especially glucose. Insulin production by beta cells begins with the cell first manufacturing a larger-than-insulin protein called *proinsulin*. This is then broken down to *insulin* and a left-over molecule called the C-peptide. Both insulin and C-peptide are stored in the cell and are released into the circulation in response to stimulation. C-peptide has no known effect. Insulin circulating in the blood reacts with specific cell membrane sites called *receptor sites* (see CELLS) and modifies the membrane to allow the uptake of glucose.

Insulin is the primary hormone regulating blood glucose levels by controlling the rate glucose is utilised by muscle fat, and liver cells. It acts primarily to promote the uptake of glucose, to stimulate glycogen synthesis, and to suppress the production of glucose. Insulin is needed for the cellular function of heart and other muscles, but not for the cells of the nervous system, red blood cells, intestinal mucosa, liver cells, and kidney tubules.

Most people produce 20 to 40 units of insulin daily; however, the diabetic either has no insulin at all, and is therefore insulin dependent, or does not have enough effective insulin for his needs. The insulin-dependent diabetic must receive his insulin exogenously, that is, by injection. Other diabetics can control their diabetes with diet alone, or with diet and oral hypoglycaemic agents. In early diabetes, and especially in the obese diabetic, there is often an excess of insulin, but for reasons not entirely clear, much of this insulin is not available for use because it cannot get into the cells. Another problem in the obese is that the release of insulin may be delayed after a meal, and when it is finally released it comes in a rush and in too large a quantity. When obesity is the major problem, weight reduction vastly improves blood glucose levels, and may even eliminate all symptoms of diabetes. See WEIGHT.

Body fat, therefore, appears to be a serious insulin antagonist – an element that works against insulin. Other insulin antagonists are glucagon, growth hormone, and adrenaline. There is some evidence that in certain individuals the beta cells literally 'wear out' trying to produce large amounts of insulin, which is rendered less effective by various antagonists.

Insulin was first developed in an unmodified clear form, crystalline zinc insulin, now called soluble insulin. Soluble insulin is short-acting, so to prevent the necessity of three or four injections a day, chemicals were added to insulin to prolong its action. Insulin is made from the pancreases of cattle (beef, or bovine, insulin) and pigs (pork, or porcine, insulin).

To date, artificial or synthetic insulin is not in use, but there is hope that human insulin can be synthesised by cloning bacteria (see RESEARCH). Allergies to insulin may then be decreased. When first taking insulin, many people experience insulin allergy for a few weeiks. This is evidenced by burning, redness, or swelling around the injection sites. Serious allergies to insulin are rare, but sometimes a change to pure beef or pure pork insulin is the answer. Pork insulin is chemically the closest to human insulin. See also ALLERGY.

Dosage   Treatment with insulin is a highly individual matter, and no attempt is made in this manual to suggest which insulin, how much, or what combinations are best for an individual. However, since the most common error made in the treatment of diabetes by physicians is the prescribing of too much insulin, you can assist the doctor tremendously by keeping careful records of urine tests for glucose and acetone (see URINE TESTS), noting the times of day you may have a hypoglycaemic reaction, if any, the amount of exercise taken and, of course, by keeping your weight down and following the prescribed diet.

Types of Insulin   The different forms of insulin, insulin mixtures, and possible insulin schedules are discussed here. It is suggested that you also read the entries INSULIN SYRINGES AND THEIR CARE and INSULIN INJECTIONS AND INJECTION SITES, very carefully. For further information, ask your doctor, and since one often tends to feel pressed for time in the doctor's surgery or during hospital visits, it is a good idea to list on paper any questions, and to take your record book with you. *It cannot be emphasised enough that the diabetic is the person most responsible for his care.*

A unit of insulin is a way of measuring insulin. Insulin comes in 10 cc vials in different concentrations. Insulin is made in different strengths. Most are available as 40 and 80 units per cc but soluble in the additional strength of 20 units per cc. In the future, 100 units per cc (U100) may replace all these. The colour coding of insulin which has been widely used, is now being phased out. The amount of insulin per unit remains the same; it is only the concentration in the solution that changes. This concept is sometimes hard to grasp, and even nurses who are not used to working with diabetics can become confused. (Nurses should always double-check insulin doses with another nurse before administering insulin to a patient.) The advantages of U100 insulin is that it is in line with the conversion of the metric system, and larger doses can be given in a smaller amount of fluid, which is important in subcutaneous injections.

All vials of insulin bear an expiration date, and they should not be used after that date.

Soluble Insulin

Appearance – clear, colourless liquid

Action – rapid onset ½ to 1 hour

Peak of action – 2 to 4 hours

Duration of action – 4 to 6 hours

Time of administration – 15 to 20 minutes before breakfast or as ordered by your doctor.

Because the action of soluble insulin is more like the natural action of the body's own insulin supplied by the pancreas, some doctors are suggesting that diabetics give themselves an injection of soluble insulin before each meal. Some may require a small amount of NPH or Lente insulin added to the presupper dose, and then followed later by a bedtime snack. This method offers better control of blood glucose, and perhaps fewer complications of diabetes in later years. Dr Peter Forsham of the University of California in San Francisco has been working with this concept for some time. Do this only with the approval and help of your doctor.

140

Globin Zinc Insulin
  Appearance – clear, yellowish liquid
  Action – intermediate: onset 1 to 2 hours
  Peak of action – 6 to 8 hours
  Duration of action – 12 to 14 hours
  Time of administration – ½ to 1 hour before breakfast or
    as ordered by the doctor
  Globin Zinc Insulin as an intermediate-acting insulin has
    generally been replaced by NPH and Lente insulins, but
    is still available for use. Manufactured by E. R. Squibb
    and Sons.

Lente Insulin (Insulin Zinc Suspension)
  Appearance – cloudy liquid
  Action – intermediate: onset 1 to 2 hours
  Peak of action – 6 to 8 hours
  Duration of action – up to 24 hours
  Time of administration – ½ to 1 hour before breakfast or
    as ordered by the doctor.

NPH (Neutral Protamine Hagedorn Insulin) Isophane Insulin Suspension
  Appearance – cloudy liquid
  Action – intermediate: onset 1 to 2 hours
  Peak of action – 6 to 8 hours
  Duration of action – 12 to 14 hours
  Time of administration – ½ to 1 hour before breakfast or
    as ordered by the doctor.

PZI (Protamine Zinc Insulin Suspension)
  Action – long: onset 4 to 6 hours
  Peak of action – 18 hours (plus or minus)
  Duration of action – about 24 hours
  Time of administration – 1 hour before breakfast or as
    ordered by the doctor.

Semilente Insulin (Insulin Zinc Suspension)
  Appearance – cloudy liquid
  Action – rapid: onset ½ to 1 hour
  Peak of action – 2 to 4 hours
  Duration of action – 8 to 10 hours
  Time of administration – 20 to 30 minutes before breakfast
    or as ordered by the doctor.

Ultralente Insulin (Extended Insulin Zinc Suspension)
> Appearance – cloudy liquid
> Action – long: onset 4 to 6 hours
> Peak of action – 8 to 12 hours
> Duration of action – up to 36 hours
> Time of administration – 1 hour before breakfast or as ordered by the doctor.

Insulin Mixtures Combinations of two insulins are readily mixed when they are needed, and when basic rules are followed. U100 Insulin can be diluted with sterile normal saline, when very small doses are required for small children; for example, ½ U100 insulin and ½ normal saline makes a mixture that contains 50 units per cc, or U50 insulin. Further dilutions can be made this way. A tuberculin syringe (see INSULIN SYRINGES AND THEIR CARE) is usually used to measure very small doses of U100 insulin and its diluted forms, because this syringe holds 1 cc of fluid as does the U100 syringe.

Soluble insulin may be mixed with NPH insulin in any amount, but it must be used right away. Soluble insulin may also be mixed with Lente insulin if the amount of soluble insulin is not greater than the amount of Lente. Soluble insulin can be mixed with PZI insulin and can be mixed ahead of time. Semilente, Ultralente, and Lente can be mixed together in any combination and can be mixed ahead of time.

Two-Dose Schedule With such a variety of insulins and insulin mixtures available, it would seem that a mixture might easily be found that would serve the needs of each individual; however, as already mentioned, each person is different in his response to his diabetes, his diet, exercise habits, and response to stress. The times given for the onset, peaks, and durations of actions of insulin are only averages, so when logic would indicate that Ultralente in the correct dosage would cover your needs for a whole day, the facts are that a 24 to 36-hour coverage may overlap so much that one might get a reaction sometime during the second day. One answer for diabetics requiring 30 or more units of insulin per day is to give soluble insulin with one of the intermediate acting insulins. A common way of working this out is to give two-thirds of a dose in the morning and one-third before supper. Soluble insulin can be combined with both doses, or a small dose of intermediate-acting NPH or Lente given before supper. Careful records will help the doctor monitor your insulin needs.

Filling the Syringe Mixing two insulins together requires concentration and understanding of the principles involved. Assume you are to mix 10 units of soluble insulin with 30 units of NPH insulin. Most doctors will tell you to draw up the soluble insulin into the syringe first; this means you will first have to inject air into the NPH vial. (If air is not injected into an airtight vial equal to the amount of fluid to be withdrawn, a vaccum is created making it difficult to withdraw the fluid – this becomes increasingly so as the vial empties.) Wash your hands and wipe both vial tops with an alcohol swab. Draw air into the syringe to the 30-unit mark (equal volume of air to NPH insulin) and inject the air into the NPH vial. Withdraw the needle, and draw more air into the syringe; this time, draw air to the 10-unit mark, the number of units of soluble insulin you need. Inject this air into the soluble insulin vial, but do not withdraw the needle; instead, very carefully pull out (aspirate) the soluble insulin to the 10-unit mark on the syringe. You now have 10 units of soluble insulin in the syringe. If there are any bubbles, pull out more insulin and inject the bubbles back into the bottle, but be sure you ultimately have 10 units. Withdraw the needle.

Since the NPH insulin is a modified insulin and is cloudy, mix it well by rolling (not shaking) the vial between the hands. (Shaking the vial produces bubbles, which you want to avoid.) Place the needle into the rubber stopper of the NPH insulin vial. *Do not inject the soluble insulin into the NPH vial.* Instead, carefully draw out 30 units of NPH insulin. Since you already have 10 units of soluble insulin in the syringe, you will need to pull the plunger back to the 40-unit mark on the syringe. Any bubbles may be eliminated by tapping the barrel of the syringe with a finger; but carefully; *there should be no bubbles.* Do not insert the needle above the line of fluid in the vial, since this will deliver air into the syringe. Practice makes perfect; carelessness and inattention produce mistakes. WARNING: Patients who mix two types of insulin must not change the order of mixing prescribed by the physician, nor change the model or brand of syringe and needle without first consulting a physician or pharmacist. Failure to heed this warning can result in an error in insulin dosage. See also DRUGS, STORAGE OF; INSULIN INJECTION AND INJECTION SITES; INSULINE SYRINGES AND THEIR CARE; SLIDING-SCALE INSULIN COVERAGE.

INSULIN ANTAGONISTS Elements, such as drugs, or hormones, which work against insulin, thus indirectly inhibiting the metabolism of glucose. Major insulin antagonists are glucagon, somatostatin, growth hormone, cortisol (hydrocortisone), epinephrine (adrenaline), and body fat. See WEIGHT.

INSULIN ATROPHY See INSULIN INJECTION AND INJECTION SITES.

INSULIN BLOOD LEVELS See IMMUNOASSAY.

INSULIN COMA See HYPOGLYCAEMIC REACTIONS.

INSULIN COMBINATIONS See Insulin Mixtures and Mixing Bottle or Vial under INSULIN.

INSULIN DEPENDENT The diabetic who must have insulin injections. See also DIABETES MELLITUS.

INSULIN DOSAGE See Dosage and Two-Dose Schedule, under INSULIN.

INSULIN HYPERSECRETION See IV Glucagon Test and IV Tolbutamide (Orinase) Test under BLOOD TESTS.

INSULIN INFUSION Soluble insulin can be infused continuously into a vein using an intravenous drip, a procedure used in hospitals.

INSULIN INJECTION AND INJECTION SITES See also INSULIN SYRINGES AND THEIR CARE. Insulin can be injected in many areas of the body, but certain precautions should be followed: Do not inject insulin at the midline of the back or abdomen because of nerve patterns. There is evidence that when insulin is injected into the thigh of a person who then goes out to run, it may be utilised faster than if it had been injected in another area. It is generally agreed that insulin is absorbed more slowly from fat tissue than from muscle tissue, and most rapidly intravenously.

Insulin is usually given subcutaneously, under the skin

ROTATION SITES FOR THE INJECTION OF INSULIN
(This is an extreme example, rotation on the thighs is often adequate)

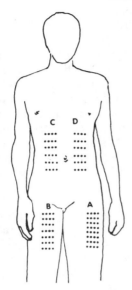
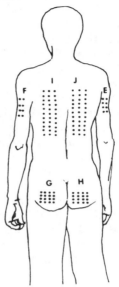

Use a schedule of injections so that at least 30 days pass before the same site is reused. Make an injection chart for each area of the body. You can copy the one at right by hand or by duplicating machine.

Label each chart with the area being used – left thigh, or right shoulder, for example. Note the date in the next empty circle each time you get an injection. The arrows indicate a suggested rotation pattern; actually any pattern could be used. Keep the current chart with the syringes so that it will always be handy when you need it. Save the marked charts until you have used all the injection sites and are ready to begin the rotation pattern over again.

INJECTION CHART
Area Being Used:

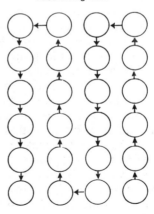

145

into fat tissue, or preferably into a pocket between the fat layer and the muscle layer. The area to be injected is cleansed with an alcohol swab and elevated by grasping the tissues between the thumb and fingers. A variety of techniques have been suggested concerning the angle of the needle. Some feel the needle should be injected straight down into the tissue at a 90° angle, while others insist that an angle of 45° or less is more effective in reaching the desired pocket. Actually, it may take some experimentation for each person to discover where the pocket is and what length of needle is needed to reach it. This pocket differs not only from person to person but from one area of the body to another. An example of this is a person who has heavy, muscular thighs but a lean abdomen. A 1-inch needle may be perfect for the heavy thigh, while a ½-inch needle is more suited to injection sites on the abdomen and back. See Filling the Syringe under INSULIN.

Once the technique of injection is mastered and the needle is in the pocket, pull back on the plunger (aspirate). If blood appears in the syringe, the end of the needle is in a vein and the insulin must not be injected (insulin works too quickly when given intravenously). Withdraw the needle and reinject in a area one or two fingers' width away. If there is a slight oozing of blood after the needle has been withdrawn, this does not mean insulin has been injected into a vein, but that a vein has been pierced. Wipe the area with the alcohol swab; it should stop bleeding shortly, although you may need to apply a bandaid. (If you bleed often and get black-and-blue spots, notify your doctor; aspirin or other drugs may be the cause.) If, on withdrawal of the needle, insulin leaks out of the injection site, try holding the needle in the tissues for about 10 seconds before withdrawal. This is not painful and usually is effective. A method of injection called the 'Z-track technique' is effective in preventing the leakage of drugs injected into the tissue. This technique requires practice and skill, but anyone who has a problem with insulin leakage, which does not respond to the method of leaving the needle in the injection site as described above, will find it worthwhile to consult with a doctor or nurse.

146

Lipodystrophy A disturbance involving the tissues into which insulin is injected; it includes atrophy, or pitting, and hypertrophy, or swelling. In the past, insulin was less pure than today's product. Not only did this impurity cause allergies (see ALLERGY; INSULIN), but it was probably responsible in part for the lipodystrophies at injection sites. Using cold insulin may also have been responsible (see DRUGS, STORAGE OF); however, the most frequent cause of lipodystrophies is the repeated injection of insulin in one site. When the same injection site is used repeatedly, the tissue tends to become less sensitive to the needle, and the injection is less painful. Repeated injection in one site can render insulin less effective because of poor absorption from overinjected areas. A method of injecting small amounts of insulin to these areas as a corrective procedure is controversial. If you have this problem, consult with your doctor.

Rotation of Injection Sites The site of insulin injection must be changed with each injection. This is made easy by using a chart such as the one shown on page 145.

INSULINOMA See TUMOURS.

INSULINOPOENIA Less insulin than normal.

INSULIN PILLS Insulin does not come in pill form. See ORAL HYPOGLYCAEMIC AGENTS; RESEARCH.

INSULIN REACTION See HYPOGLYCAEMIC REACTIONS.

INSULIN RECEPTORS See CELLS.

INSULIN RESISTANT DIABETES Insulin resistance exists when 200 or more units of insulin are required for more than two consecutive days when no acidosis or infection is present. There are two types of insulin resistance: (1) immune insulin resistance, which is rare, the result of the action of antibodies on insulin, making it unavailable for use (see ALLERGY); and (2) nonimmune insulin resistance, which is most commonly caused by obesity (see WEIGHT). See also DIABETES MELLITUS.

INSULIN SHOCK See HYPOGLYCAEMIC REACTIONS.

INSULIN STORAGE See DRUGS, STORAGE OF.

INSULIN SYRINGES AND THEIR CARE A syringe consists of a barrel with a plunger to push the contents through a needle. Several types of syringes are specially made for the

147

injection of insulin; they must be prescribed by a doctor.

Disposable Plastic Syringes Increasingly popular, these come presterilised in paper or plastic packages with very sharp 26- or 27-gauge ½" or ⅝" needles attached. If you mix two types of insulin, do not change the type of syringe without the approval of the doctor or pharmacist (see Insulin Mixtures under INSULIN). The disposable syringes described here have been designed to eliminate 'dead space', which refers to a small amount of insulin left in the hub of the syringe at the area of needle attachment after injection. Becton Dickinson Co. (B-D Plastipak) and Sherwood Medical Industries (Monoject) make 1 cc insulin syringes.

Reusable Glass Syringes These syringes can be ordered in a variety of sizes and can be used with either disposable or reusable needles. Most common is the 1 cc size made to British Standard 1619. Glass syringes, if not broken, are less expensive over a period of time. But because they require special care they are less convenient for travelling. Glass syringes must be sterilised after purchase, before use. To sterilise you may wrap the syringe parts in foil and bake in a preheated oven at 350°F for 15 to 20 minutes. Or you may boil them in water, as follows:

Prepare a pan with a basket strainer that fits inside it, and place the syringe parts in the strainer. If the needle is the reusable type, place the needle in the strainer also, and cover with water – preferably distilled water. (Do not use hard water, or water that is heavily chlorinated, because this causes mineral deposits that may obscure the markings of the syringe, and can, in time, make the operation of the syringe difficult. If soft water is not available, add 1 tablespoon of vinegar or baking soda to the water.) Place a cover on the pan, bring the water to a boil and simmer for 15 minutes. Remove the strainer from the pan, pour off the water, replace the strainer in the empty pan and allow the syringe parts to cool. Then reassemble and place in a storage container filled with alcohol. (To do this, tie a string or thread around the top of the barrel and immerse the syringe in the alcohol.) Before using the syringe, push the plunger back and forth to expel any alochol.

The storage container must also be sterilised: Wash it

with soap and water, rinse and fill with boiling water; let stand for about five minutes, then pour off the water (use a pot-holder!) To keep the syringe sterile, fill the storage container with 70 per cent isopropyl alcohol. Ordinary methylated spirit is satisfactory if it does not contain glycerin. For the few persons who are sensitive to this alcohol, try 91 per cent alcohol; if this too is irritating, boil or bake the syringe daily. In any case, the container must be sterilised once a week.

Tuberculin Syringes   There are made in the 1 cc size and have a smaller bore than the insulin syringe, making it possible to measure insulin with greater accuracy. They are sometimes used to give very small doses of insulin to babies and small children. These syringes are marked in divisions of ten, as is the 100-unit insulin syringe, and can be used only with U100 insulin.

Automatic Syringes   Sold under such names as Medijector and Jet-spray. They are expensive and are not generally recommended for use with insulin because it is difficult to obtain accurate measurement with them.

A syringe which makes one click per division on the glass may be helpful. Alternatively, a stop may be put on the plunger, so that it can draw up a pre-set number of units and no more (a 'blocked' syringe).

Needles   Needles for injection are available in a variety of sizes. B-D Plastipak needles are ½ inch, 26 gauge, while Monoject needles are ½ inch, 27 gauge. (The larger the number of gauge, the smaller the diameter of the needle.) Both needles are very sharp and do not detach from the syringe. For some diabetics these needles may not be long enough for injection into areas where there is a thick layer of fat over the muscles. Both disposable and reusable needles can be purchased when a longer needle is required and then can be used with both glass syringes or disposable syringes. See also INSULIN INJECTION AND INJECTION SITES.

INSULIN – TRAVELLING WITH   See TRAVELLING WITH DIABETES.

INSULIN TUMOUR   Insulinoma. See TUMOURS.

INSULIN ZINC SUSPENSION   Lente insulin. See IN-SULIN.

INSURANCE   Life insurance is available to most diabetics between the ages of 15 and 65 at reasonable rates, and sometimes at standard rates. Most companies will require a medical examination and will ask for a report from your diabetic specialist.

For automobile insurance, see DRIVING. See also SOCIAL SECURITY BENEFITS.

INTAKE AND OUTPUT   Intake: All fluids taken by mouth, nasogastric tube, and intravenously (IV), are measured and recorded. Output: All fluids removed from the body are measured, including urine and vomitus; if the patient is sweating profusely, or has diarrhoea, the amount is estimated. All measurements are recorded every 12 hours, and totalled and recorded every 24 hours. A doctor usually orders intake and output procedures; however, they are also initiated by a nurse when she feels the patient is retaining or losing fluid. Urine outputs may be measured as often as every ½ hour when there is a question of kidney function or severe dehydration.

INTENSIVE CARE UNIT (ICU)   A section of a hospital for patients who need care by specially trained medical personnel, utilising special equipment.

INTERCOURSE   See SEXUAL INTERCOURSE.

INTERMEDIATE-ACTING INSULINS   Globin, Lente, and NPH insulins. See INSULIN.

INTERMEDIC, INC.   See TRAVELLING WITH DIABETES.

INTERMITTENT CLAUDICATION   See LEG PAIN.

INTERN   A medical doctor (MD) continuing training in a hospital for one or two years following graduation from medical school. In the United States internship is required for all medical doctors. In the UK, the name house physician or houseman is used.

INTERNATIONAL ASSOCIATION FOR MEDICAL ASSISTANCE TO TRAVELLERS (IAMAT)   See TRAVELLING WITH DIABETES.

INTERNATIONAL DIABETES FEDERATION (IDF)   See TRAVELLING WITH DIABETES.

INTERNATIONAL LUGGAGE REGISTRY   See TRAVELLING WITH DIABETES.

INTERNIST   A specialist – a medical doctor who has had

training in internal medicine. Most doctors treating diabetes are internists. See also DIABETOLOGIST; ENDOCRINOLOGIST.

INTEROSSEOUS WASTING The wasting (atrophy) of the muscles and ligaments between bones, and especially between the thumb and index finger. Since severe diabetes rarely goes untreated these days, this complication is not frequently observed.

INTESTINES Part of digestive tract. The small intestine consists of three parts: the duodenum, the jejunum, and the ileum. The largest intestine consists of the caecum (with the appendix), the colon, and the rectum. See also DIABETIC NEUROPATHY.

INTRACELLULAR WATER See CELLS.

INTRADERMAL INJECTION The injection of substances just into or under the skin, but not into the layers under the skin (subcutaneous). Intradermal injections make a blister or a bubble. Insulin is not well absorbed from this type of injection. See also INSULIN INJECTION AND INJECTION SITES.

INTRAMUSCULAR INJECTION (IM) The injection of substances into the muscles. To prevent damage to the nerves, IM injections should be given only by persons trained to do them properly. Insulin is given IM at times by doctors and nurses for faster action. If you think you have given yourself an injection in the muscle, be alert for possible hypoglycaemic reaction. See also INSULIN INJECTION AND INJECTION SITES.

INTRA-OCULAR LENSES See EYESIGHT.

INTRA-UTERINE DEVICE (IUD) See CONTRACEPTIVES.

INTRAVENOUS INFUSION (IV) The administration of substances into a vein. This can be a single dose, or a continuous infusion (drip) from an IV bottle. Insulin is sometimes given this way in the hospital.

INTRAVENOUS PYELOGRAM (IVP) A special X-ray test of kidney function in which radiopaque dye is injected into the blood stream.

INULIN See POLYSACCHARIDES.

IN VITRO In glass. Refers to studies performed in the

laboratory under artifical conditions, usually in a test tube.

IN VIVO   In life. Refers to studies performed in the living organism.

ION   See ELECTROLYTES.

ISCHAEMIA   A temporary lack of blood supply usually caused by pressure on a blood vessel as a result of being poorly positioned in bed or remaining too long in one position, or by ill-fitting clothing, casts, or round garters. See also BED SORES.

ISLETS OF LANGERHANS   (also called **Islands of Langerhans**)   See PANCREAS.

ISOPHANE INSULIN SUSPENSION   NPH insulin. See INSULIN.

ISOPROPYL ALCOHOL   Rubbing alcohol. See also ALCOHOL; ALCOHOL SWABS.

ITALIAN DIABETIC DIET   See FOOD EXCHANGES, Exchange Lists for Ethnic Foods.

ITCHING   Irritation of the skin. Severe itching is called pruritus, or urticaria. Scratching may open the skin to infection and should be avoided.

IUD   Intra-uterine device. See CONTRACEPTIVES.

IV   See INTRAVENOUS INFUSION.

IV GLUCAGON TEST   See BLOOD TESTS.

IV GLUCOSE TOLERANCE TEST (IV-GTT)   Intravenous glucose tolerance test. See BLOOD TESTS.

IVP   See INTRAVENOUS PYELOGRAM.

IV TOLBUTAMIDE (Orinase) TEST   See BLOOD TESTS.

J

JAUNDICE An excess of bilibrubin in the system, often first seen as yellowish colouring of the whites of the eyes, followed by a yellow cast to the skin, dark brownish urine, and light-coloured stools. Jaundice is not a disease in itself but is an indication of disease. There is a possibility that oral hypoglycaemic agents can cause jaundice in susceptible diabetics. If you have any of these symptoms, consult with the doctor immediately. See Bilirubin under BILE; LIVER.

JET LAG See TRAVELLING WITH DIABETES.

JET SPRAY An automatic syringe. See INSULIN SYRINGES AND THEIR CARE.

JOBS FOR DIABETICS See EMPLOYMENT.

JOINT PAIN See CHARCOT JOINTS.

JOULES A term for the energy supplied by food. It is used in place of the word calorie. There are 4.18 joules in each calorie; therefore, a food item that contains 300 joules contains about 70 calories. (The figure is obtained by dividing 300 by 4.18.) See FOOD EXCHANGES.

JUNK FOOD Food with little or no nutritional value; it often has a high content of sugar or carbohydrates. Sweets are largely junk food, as are soda pop (tonic) and potato chips. Sugar provides energy, but no vitamins or minerals.

JUVENILE DIABETES MELLITUS See DIABETES MELLITUS, JUVENILE-ONSET.

K

KCAL or KCALORIES   The energy of heat required to raise 1 kilogram (2.2 pounds) of water 1 degree C. See also CALORIE; METRIC SYSTEM.

KETOACIDOSIS   See DIABETIC KEOTACIDOSIS.

KETO-DIASTIX   See URINE TESTS.

KETOGENESIS   The production of ketone bodies. See below.

KETONAEMIA   Ketone bodies in the blood. See KETONE BODIES; KETOSIS.

KETONE BODIES (Ketones)   Confusion may exist when the word 'ketone' is used interchangeably with acetone. Acetone is a ketone body, the one most commonly measured in the home testing of urine with reagent strips and tablets (see URINE TESTS). There are two other ketone bodies, however: acetoacetic acid (also called diacetic acid) and beta-hydroxybutyric acid, or B-hydroxybutyric acid. These are all chemical compounds produced in the liver and transported to the tissues where they are utilised as fat for energy. Normally the concentration of ketones in the blood is very low and not present in the urine at all. In severe diabetes, when the blood glucose is high but not available to the cells because of the lack of effective insulin, fat stores from the tissues are made available for energy at a rate greater than they can be used. In diabetic ketoacidosis, in other conditions of impaired carbohydrate metabolism, and in starvation states, ketone bodies also accumulate. This leads to ketosis, or ketonaemia, an excess of ketone bodies in the blood. Ketone bodies are then excreted in the urine, a condition called ketonuria; if the concentration of ketones is high enough, the breath smells 'fruity' like nail polish and can even be mistaken for the odour of alcohol. This is called acetone breath. Caught in time, the administration of insulin and glucose will restore ketone bodies to a normal concentration, and correct the acid state of the body. See

154

also ACIDOSIS; DIABETIC KETOACIDOSIS; KREBS CYCLE.

KETONURIA   Ketone bodies in the urine. See KETONE BODIES.

KETOSIS   Ketone bodies in the blood. Ketosis is a warning sign that the body has broken down fats in an attempt to get fuel. Adverse reactions in the diabetic include dehydration and the development of an acid condition of the blood. In extreme cases coma or unconsciousness may occur. See also KETONE BODIES.

KETOSIS-PRONE DIABETES   See DIABETES MELLITUS, JUVENILE-ONSET.

KETOSTIX   See URINE TESTS.

KIDNEY DISEASE (Nephropathy)   (See also KIDNEYS.) The nature and process of kidney disease in relation to diabetes are not clearly understood. There are no firm studies that show a relationship between nephropathy and high blood glucose, but until this is ruled out, it is felt that for the sake of healthy kidneys, the blood glucose should be kept as near normal levels as possible. This becomes increasingly difficult to maintain as kidney disease increases and the renal threshold increases; in this case, urine tests become a less reliable test of blood glucose level. See also RENAL THRESHOLD.

There is more than one disease process in kidney disease. One is the Kimmelsteil-Wilson lesion, thought by many to be a scarring or thickening of the glomeruli (capillaries) of the kidneys; another is the thickening of the basement cell membranes of the nephrons (the main functioning units of the kidneys). Both can seriously affect the filtering of the blood, which is the primary function of the kidney, causing the kidney eventually to fail completely. When the blood is not filtered, little or no urine is produced (conditions called respectively oliguria and anuria) with the result that nitrogenous compounds (urea, creatinine, and uric acid) from the breakdown of protein accumulate in the blood (azotaemia) and progress to general toxic condition called uraemia, which includes azotaemia and acid-base imbalance.

Infection and inflammation of the kidneys is more common in the diabetic than in the nondiabetic.

Pyelonephritis, most often caused by bacteria originating through the bladder, is hard to control; nephritis, or Bright's disease, is an inflammation and degeneration of the filtering ability of the glomerulus and has nothing to do with diabetes.

Examination of the Kidneys In renal biopsy, a needle is inserted into the kidney, and tissue is removed for examination. Nephrotomography is a method used with or without radiopaque dye to visualise kidney tissue in layers; renal angiography is a method of injecting radiopaque dye into the blood stream and taking X-rays to check the condition of the renal arteries. In retrograde radiography, radiopaque dye is injected through a catheter (see) into the ureter and then X-rayed to check for obstructions.

Blood tests for kidney function include blood urea, albumin, and creatinine (see BLOOD TESTS). Urine tests for kidney function, especially the creatinine clearance test, are to be found under URINE TESTS.

Dialysis When the kidneys shut down and fluids and waste products collect in the body in spite of treatment with drugs, there are two courses of action that may be followed: one is to try to find a suitable kidney for transplantation and the other is to use dialysis.

Peritoneal dialysis has been used primarily in acute kidney failure, but is favoured over haemodialysis by some patients because they feel better in the periods between treatments. A tube is inserted through the abdominal wall and peritoneum, and a special solution is run through the tube into the abdominal cavity. The peritoneum, a thin tissue lining the abdominal cavity, acts as a filter and by osmosis, the metabolic wastes are drained off, removing toxic substances and re-establishing fluid and electrolyte balance.

Haemodialysis is used more often to treat chronic kidney failure. A dialysis machine is connected to the patient's bloodstream, accomplishing the same chemical exchanges, described above under peritoneal dialysis. Dialysis is not painful, but it is time-consuming and tedious, taking several hours to complete, and must be repeated as often as several times a week. See also ELECTROLYTES;

KIDNEYS; OSMOSIS; RESEARCH.

KIDNEY MACHINE (for Haemodialysis) See KIDNEY DISEASE.

KIDNEYS Part of the urinary system. There are two kidneys; each one is connected by a ureter to the urinary bladder, which collects urine and passes it out of the body through the urethra. The adult kidney is about 4.5 inches (11.43 cm) long; each is capped by a small endocrine gland called the adrenal. The kidneys are located at the back of the body, just above the waist – one on each side of the spinal column. The function of the kidneys is to filter wastes from the blood, transforming them into urine and eliminating them from the body in order to prevent a toxic build-up. The waste products are derived mainly from the breakdown of food and body tissues in normal wear and tear. The kidneys are of major importance in maintaining the acid-base balance in the body, by eliminating or conserving salts and water. When blood glucose levels rise above normal, the kidneys filter out some of the excess glucose into the urine. However, when there is a high renal threshold, large amounts of glucose remain in the blood; in this instance a urine test for glucose does not adequately indicate true blood glucose levels.

The blood reaches the kidneys through the large abdominal artery, called the abdominal aorta, branching to each kidney by way of the renal arteries, and entering the nephrons through a tuft of capillaries called the glomerulus. The main functioning unit of the kidney is called the *nephron*; each kidney has about 1,000,000 nephrons. The kidneys handle about 1,100 to 1,200 ml of blood each minute – about a fourth of the output of the heart per minute. Any condition or disease inhibiting or preventing the proper functioning of any part of the kidney can be critical to the body as a whole. See also KIDNEY DISEASE; URINARY BLADDER; URINE.

KIDNEY TRANSPLANTS See RESEARCH.

KILOCALORIE See CALORIE; KCALORIE.

KILOGRAM See METRIC SYSTEM.

KIMMELSTIEL-WILSON DISEASE See KIDNEY DISEASE.

KREBS CYCLE Named after Hans Krebs, a British biochemist, this is a series of reactions that most cells use to convert nutrient substances into the energy they use to perform their functions in the body. It is also known as the citric acid cycle because the first molecule in the cycle is citric acid. Oxygen is needed in these reactions, and the final waste products are water and carbon dioxide.

The key starting compound in the Krebs cycle is acetyl coenzyme A, which is also involved in the manufacture of fatty acids and cholesterol. In diabetes mellitus, acetyl coenzyme A is not used normally and accumulates, reacting to form acetoacetyl coenzyme A. It is the breakdown of acetoacetyl coenzyme A that yields acetone. See also BIOSYNTHESIS; KETONE BODIES; METABOLISM.

KUSSMAUL'S RESPIRATIONS See AIR HUNGER; DIABETIC KETOACIDOSIS.

L

LABELS   See NUTRITIONAL LABELLING.

LABIA   See GENITALIA.

LABILE DIABETES   Diabetes that is hard to control. See also DIABETES MELLITUS, JUVENILE-ONSET.

LABORATORY TESTS   Tests done by the laboratory as ordered by the doctor. See individual tests; BLOOD TESTS; URINE TESTS.

LACTATE   Salt from lactic acid (which see).

LACTATION   See PREGNANCY AND CHILDBIRTH.

LACTIC ACID (Lactate)   In the living cell, one of the breakdown processes of glycogen or glucose yields lactic acid. This process, which requires no oxygen, frees energy rapidly. A muscle that has contracted many times, and used up its stores of organic phosphates and glycogen, has consequently accumulated lactic acid; it is unable to contract any more and is said to be fatigued (sore muscles). Fatigue is primarily induced by this accumulation of lactic acid.

LACTIC ACIDOSIS   (also called **Lactacidosis** and **Lactate Acidosis**)   A type of metabolic acidosis caused by too much lactate in the body. One of the oral hypoglycaemic agents Phenformin HC1, a biguanide, can cause lactic acidosis in some diabetics, even though this complication is rare. Lactic acidosis can be a complication in diabetic ketoacidosis, and in liver or kidney disease. It is also seen in drug poisoning, especially from salicylates (including aspirin); prolonged vomiting; heart failure; acute alcoholism, especially if the patient has not been eating; and other diseases. Dehydration is usually present, hyperventilation, stupor or coma may exist. In lactic acidosis that is not a complication of diabetic ketoacidosis, the blood glucose may be normal or even low, and acidosis as measured with Acetest tablets (see URINE TESTS) will not show up because the acid involved is not acetone. See also KETONE BODIES.

Dialysis (see under KIDNEY DISEASE) may be instituted as treatment for lactic acidosis. See also METABOLIC ACIDOSIS.

LACTOGEN   Any substance that stimulates the flow of milk. See PREGNANCY AND CHILDBIRTH.

LACTO-OVO-VEGETARIAN DIET   A vegetarian diet that utilises eggs and milk. See Vegetarian Food Exchanges under FOOD EXCHANGES.

LACTOSE   Milk sugar. See PREGNANCY AND CHILDBIRTH; SUGAR.

LANGERHANS   In 1869 Paul Langerhans, a German medical student, discovered the special cells in the pancreas that were later named after him: the islets of Langerhans.

LASER BEAM   See RETINA; RETINOPATHY.

LARGE BABIES   See FAT BABIES; PREGNANCY AND CHILDBIRTH.

LATENT DIABETES MELLITUS   See Classification of Diabetes under DIABETES MELLITUS; PREGNANCY AND CHILDBIRTH.

LATE-ONSET DIABETES   See DIABETES MELLITUS, ADULT-ONSET.

LATERAL   On or toward the side of the body.

LAXATIVES   Any medicine, herb, or food that loosens the bowels and helps in the evacuation of faeces (stool). A simple thing such as drinking one or two glasses of water right after getting up and before breakfast may help relieve constipation. Exercise of any kind helps, because it keeps the whole body in better condition. Fibre, or roughage, is important in maintaining good elimination. See FIBRE.

LEGAL BLINDNESS   See BLINDNESS.

LEG PAIN   Pain after walking or exercise, usually in the legs, rarely in the arms, can be caused by the narrowing of the arteries because of atherosclerosis or by damage to the nerves serving the leg muscles. The pain is relieved by rest. Claudication is a word for pain, and leg pain of this type is often referred to as intermittent claudication. It usually affects the toes first, then spreads to the legs. Sometimes it affects only one leg. It occurs most often in elderly males. Pain that occurs at rest usually indicates a more severe blockage of the arteries, and this pain may be relieved by walking. Sudden, severe leg pain while at rest indicates the

160

complete blockage of an artery. Call the doctor immediately or go to the nearest hospital.

LEGUMES   They include dried beans of all kinds, dried peas, lentils, and chick-peas (garbanzos). Soybeans are especially valuable as a source of vegetable protein. See also FOOD EXCHANGES, Lists 4 and 5, and Vegetarian Food Exchanges.

LENS OF THE EYE   See EYESIGHT.

LENTE INSULIN (Insulin Zinc Suspension)   See INSULIN.

LESION   A change or alteration on the skin or in the body that is not supposed to be there can be called a lesion. Tumours are often called lesions.

LEUKOCYTES   White blood cells. See BLOOD; THYMUS GLAND.

LEVELS OF CONSCIOUSNESS   See COMA.

LEVULOSE   See SUGAR.

LICENCE TO DRIVE   See DRIVING.

LIFE INSURANCE   See INSURANCE.

LIGHT-HEADEDNESS   Low blood glucose may be the cause. See HYPOGLYCAEMIC REACTIONS.

LIGHT COAGULATION   Photocoagulation. See RETINA, RETINOPATHY.

LINOLEIC ACID   A fatty acid. See LIPIDS.

LIPAEMIA   Fat and fatlike substances in the blood. See LIPIDS.

LIPAEMIA RETINALIS   See RETINA, RETINOPATHY.

LIPIDS   Fat and fatlike substances that are insoluble in water. The principal types of compounds classified as lipids can be listed as:

1. Simple lipids, which include the fats and waxes. Neutral fats constitute 98 to 99 per cent of food and body fats and are composed of glycerol (an alcohol) and fatty acids. Triglycerides are in this group.
2. Compound lipids. These are lipids that contain fatty acids and glycerol, and an additional molecule. For example, phospholipids with a phosphate molecule, or glycolipids with a carbohydrate molecule.
3. Derived lipids are substances that are the product of lipid breakdown (hydrolysis). These include fatty acids, glycerol, steroids, and ketone bodies. Steroids

are a physiologically important class of lipids, with cholesterol being quantitatively the predominant one.

Function of Fat Fat serves to protect the organs against injury; protect the nerves; insulate the body against rapid changes of temperature; furnish calories for energy; carry the fat-soluble vitamins A, D, E, and K; and retard hunger by depressing secretions of the stomach and by slowing down its emptying into the small intestine. Fats are the most concentrated source of energy among all foods, yielding 9 calories per gram, or 270 calories per ounce. This is true of all fats, saturated, unsaturated, or polyunsaturated, regardless of whether the fat is of animal or vegetable origin, solid or liquid (oil). Fat is broken down for use by the body into fatty acids and glycerol to nourish the cells. Fat that is not needed for energy is stored as fat tissue or excreted in the faeces (see STEATORRHOEA).

Fatty Acids These circulate in the blood as free fatty acids (FFA). There are many kinds of fatty acids; butter, for example, contains about sixty different fatty acids. Fatty acids are classified as saturated, unsaturated, or polyunsaturated. Chemically they are composed of long chains of carbon atoms. All the fatty acids in nature have an even number of carbon atoms. Fatty acids with one or more double bonds between two carbon atoms were called unsaturated. The greater the degree of unsaturation, the lower the melting point. This helps to explain why animal fats (saturated) are solids and vegetable oils (unsaturated) are liquid at room temperature. One of the most important fatty acids in the diet is linoleic acid, which the body is unable to make; it is therefore called an essential fatty acid (EFA). Polyunsaturated oils from corn, safflower, cottonseed, and sesame are rich in linoleic acid. Peanut and olive oil are two other examples of unsaturated fatty acids. Coconut and other palm oils are sources of saturated fatty acids.

Hydrogenated Fats are oils changed to solid fats by the addition of hydrogen in the manufacturing process, such as is used to make margarines and vegetable shortening. If not otherwise stated, margarines and vegetable shortenings are made from coconut and palm oils, both highly saturated.

Phospholipids are important constituents of the membranes of animal cells in general and nerve cells in particular. Phospholipids aid in the blood-clotting mechanism (coagulation of blood), and act with bile salts as emulsifying agents in fat metabolism. See BILE; LIVER.

Blood Lipids most commonly measured in the clinical laboratory are cholesterol and triglycerides. Cholesterol is a hydrocarbon-like steroid compound found in animal cells. Steroid molecules display great structural similarity. The body obtains cholesterol from food, and can make cholesterol in body tissues. In the liver it is used as a raw material for building other usable steroids such as the sex hormones progesterone and testosterone and the adrenocortical hormones (see ADRENAL GLANDS). The amount of cholesterol in the body varies from person to person. Authorities do not agree on what the normal level should be. In general, 120 to 250 mg/dl of serum is an accepted range. Many doctors consider an ideal level to be below 220 mg/dl.

Foods high in cholesterol are the organ meats such as liver, kidney, and sweetbreads (brains and pancreas), egg yolk, and fish eggs (roe). Smaller amounts of cholesterol are found in whole milk, cheese made from whole milk, cream cheese, ice cream, and beef.

Hypercholesterolaemia, or a high blood cholesterol level, is found in uncontrolled diabetes, nephrosis, heart disease, and other diseases. The relationship between diabetes and high lipid levels is not clear (see BLOOD TESTS).

Triglycerides are neutral fats composed of glycerol and three fatty acids. Blood triglyceride levels are normal at 25 to 150 mg/dl. They can be elevated when too many carbohydrates are eaten, and also when alcohol is taken in excess. High triglyceride levels (hypertriglyceridaemia) can be controlled by diet, and especially by weight loss. *The body needs insulin to remove triglycerides from the blood.* When diabetes is in control and the body weight is normal, triglycerides are usually at normal or near-normal levels. See BLOOD TESTS.

Lipaemia is a general term for lipids in the blood. Cholesterol and triglycerides do not circulate in the blood alone, but in combination with albumin, one of the plasma proteins, and are then referred to as lipoproteins. Lipoproteinaemia means lipoproteins in the blood, and hyperlipoproteinaemia refers to excessive amounts of lipids in the blood. In some people, the elimination or reduction of sugar can significantly lower blood lipid levels.

LIPODYSTROPHY   See INSULIN INJECTION AND INJECTION SITES.

LIPOPROTEINAEMIA   Lipoproteins in the blood. See LIPIDS.

LIPOPROTEINS   See LIPIDS.

LIQUID DIET   See DIET.

LIQUOR   See ALCOHOL.

LITER, LITRE, L   See METRIC SYSTEMS.

LIVER   The liver is the largest gland in the body, weighing 3 to 4 pounds in the adult. It is found on a lvel with and to the right of the stomach. When a doctor pushes on the upper right side, up against the ribs, he is feeling the lower edge of the liver. The liver can be compared to a factory that performs many services for the body. These include the secretion of bile, production of plasma proteins, destruction of 'worn out' red blood cells, detoxification of substances that might be damaging to the body (such as nicotine), production of blood-clotting materials, and storage of vitamins and glycogen. It is the site of GLYCOGENESIS, GLYCOGENOLYSIS, and GLUCONEOGENESIS to maintain normal blood glucose.

Insulin is not needed to transport glucose to the liver cell, but it does affect the utilisation of glucose by decreasing the rate of glycogenolysis (glycogen breakdown), increasing the rate of glycogen production, and decreasing the rate of gluconeogenesis (new glucose formation).

LIVER DISEASE   In adult-onset diabetes (see DIABETES MELLITUS, ADULT-ONSET), no specific liver disease is identified. The incidence of liver disease such as cirrhosis is high in the diabetic. Fatty liver comes from obesity in both the diabetic and nondiabetic, and can be treated successfully with diet and weight loss if not too far advanced.

In children, an enlarged liver (hepatomegaly) is sometimes observed. Hepatomegaly with weight gain and poor growth is called Mauriac syndrome, and is said to be related to poor nutrition and overtreatment with insulin. Large livers return to normal size with a reduction in insulin, and

164

in Mauriac's syndrome, the child also responds by growing taller.

LIVING WITH DIABETES   See DIABETES MELLITUS.

LONG-ACTING CARBOHYDRATES   See STARCHES.

LONG-ACTING INSULINS   PZI (Protamine Zinc Insulin) and Ultralente Insulin.   See INSULIN.

LOSS OF FEELING   See ANAESTHESIA.

LOSS OF SLEEP   See INSOMNIA.

LOW BLOOD GLUCOSE   See HYPOGLYCAEMIA; HYPOGLYCAEMIC REACTIONS.

LOW BLOOD PRESSURE   See BLOOD PRESSURE.

LOW BLOOD SUGAR   See HYPOGLYCAEMIA; HYPO-GLYCAEMIC REACTIONS.

LOW-CALORIE DIET   A diet low in calories, prescribed by the doctor and designed to facilitate weight loss. See DIET.

LOW-FAT DIET   See DIET; FOOD EXCHANGES and Vegetarian Food Exchange under FOOD EXCHANGES.

LOW-FAT MILK   See FOOD EXCHANGES, List 1.

LOW-SALT DIET   See SODIUM.

LOW-SODIUM DIET   See SODIUM and Salt Substitutes under SODIUM.

LUGGAGE   See TRAVELLING WITH DIABETES.

LUMBAR PUNCTURE   Insertion of a needle into the spinal tissues to inject medication or to withdraw cerebrospinal fluid for laboratory examination. Spinal fluid protein may be elevated in diabetic neuropathies.

LUNCH   See DIET; FOOD EXCHANGES.

LYMPH; LYMPHATIC SYSTEM   In addition to the blood vessels, the body is supplied with a separate set of small vessels called lymphatics. They originate in the tissue space as tiny lymphatic capillaries that empty into larger vessels that finally empty into the heart. On the way to the heart, the vessels pass through lymph nodes; these are small organs that filter small particles of matter out of the lympathic fluid before it empties into the heart. Lymph nodes are populated by white blood cells called lymphocytes. The colourless fluid that flows through the lymphatics is actually overflow fluid from the tissue spaces; it is known as lymph. An important function of the lymphatics is to return proteins to the blood after they leak out of the capillaries.

The lymphatic system serves as a defence against infection and disease; thus, enlarged lymph nodes indicate the presence of infection or disease. As the lymph passes through the lymph nodes, the so-called reticuloendothelial cells digest any foreign material, such as bacteria. The system is sometimes referred to as the RE system – the reticuloendothelial system. See also ALLERGY; BLOOD.

M

MACROANGIOPATHY   See BLOOD VESSEL DISEASE.

MACROPHAGE   See White Blood Cells under BLOOD.

MACULA LUTEA   Also referred to simply as macula. See RETINA, RETINOPATHY.

MALABSORPTION   See MALNUTRITION.

MALAISE   Discomfort; a feeling of being ill.

MALNUTRITION   A state of being undernourished – lacking enough food or the right sort of food for proper growth of the body, for energy, and for the repair and maintenance of body tissues. Malnutrition can also be caused by the malabsorption of food due to diarrhoea. In undiagnosed diabetes, carbohydrate cannot be used because of the lack of insulin, and there is a large calorie loss in glycosuria (glucose in the urine). When this occurs, the body resorts to using its stored protein and fat, causing ketosis, weight loss, and weakness. See also DIABETIC NEUROPATHY; KETONE BODIES; VISCERA, VISCERAL NERVES AND DISEASE.

MALTOSE   See SUGAR.

MANNITOL   See Sugar Substitutes under SUGAR.

MANUAL LABOUR   Insulin seems to work better when the body is active. Although manual labour and exercise are not the same, some of the effects are the same. Diabetics whose work involves heavy labour must eat a diet that supplies enough calories to prevent low blood glucose. If you are working and suddenly feel weak, or have other signs of low blood glucose, stop working immediately and eat something sweet. Carry the sweet in your pocket or purse, not in the glove compartment of the car. On working days it may be necessary to eat a bigger breakfast or carry a bigger lunch, or both. The doctor may advise reducing the insulin dose. Keep careful records. If you are less active at weekends, you may have to eat less to avoid high blood glucose. See also EXERCISE/SPORTS (includes a diet for exercise); HYPO-GLYCAEMIC REACTIONS.

MAPLE SYRUP See SUGAR.

MARGARINE The kind made with polyunsaturated oils is recommended. This includes margarines made from corn, safflower, soybean, cottonseed, and sesame seed oils. See also Diet Margarine under DIETETIC FOOD; FOOD EXCHANGES, List 6; and LIPIDS.

MARRIAGE Married couples, both of whom have a history of diabetes in the family are sometimes advised not to have children; however, there has been some change in the thinking about the heredity of diabetes, and there is probably less risk than previously thought. See also HEREDITY; PREGNANCY AND CHILDBIRTH.

MATURITY-ONSET DIABETES See DIABETES MELLITUS, ADULT-ONSET.

MAURIAC SYNDROME See LIVER DISEASE.

MAYONNAISE It may be advisable to use the type made with polyunsaturated oils; see MARGARINE. For diet mayonnaise, see DIETETIC FOOD. See also FOOD EXCHANGES, List 6; LIPIDS.

MEAL PLANNING AND MEALS See DIET; FOOD EXCHANGES.

MEASLES There are two types, each caused by a virus. Rubella is German measles, which lasts for a few days. Complications can occur with both types.

   If contracted during the first three months of pregnancy, German measles can cause birth defects. No woman should become pregnant without first having been immunised against German measles, either by having had the virus or by vaccine.

   A vaccine is also available for measles. See also RESEARCH.

MEASUREMENT OF INSULIN See INSULIN; INSULIN SYRINGES AND THEIR CARE.

MEASUREMENTS See METRIC SYSTEM.

MEAT See FOOD EXCHANGES, List 5. Note meat exchanges are now in three groups: lean meat, medium-fat meat, and high-fat meat.

MEAT SUBSTITUTES, or ANALOGUES See Vegetarian Food Exchanges under FOOD EXCHANGES.

MEATUS   See GENITALIA.

MEDIAL   Down the middle – midline of the body.

MEDICAL DOCTOR (MD)   See PHYSICIAN.

MEDIC ALERT   A non-profit international clearinghouse that will accept any call from a third party for vital medical information to an emergency. To register with Medic Alert, pick up an application at a pharmacy, or write to Medic Alert Foundation. Medic Alert will provide you with a bracelet or necklace engraved with information pertaining to your condition, which you can thus carry on you at all times in case of an emergency. They are made in a small size for children and the standard size for adults. The membership fee is included in the cost of the emblem and is tax deductible. NOTE: Medic Alert recommends that diabetics wear only stainless steel, as acids in the skin may cause silver and gold to tarnish.

MEDICARE   See SOCIAL SECURITY BENEFITS.

MEDICINE   See DRUGS, STORAGE OF; INSULIN; ORAL HYPOGLYCAEMIC AGENTS.

MEDI-JECTOR   Automatic syringe. See INSULIN SYRINGES AND THEIR CARE.

MEGA-VITAMINS   Large doses of vitamins. See VITAMIN C; VITAMINS.

MELITURIA   From the Greek words *meli*, or *mel*, meaning honey and *ouron*, urine, melituria means any kind of sugar in the urine. Disease or conditions other than diabetes can cause glucose or other sugars to be present in the urine. Some of the sugars found in the urine are glucose, fructose (levulose), galactose, lactose, and maltose. Clinistix will pick up only glucose. See PREGNANCY AND CHILDBIRTH; SUGAR; URINE TESTS.

MENARCHE   Beginning of menstruation in the female. See also ADOLESCENCE.

MENOPAUSE   Change of life in the female, usually between the ages of 45 and 50, and signalled by the decreasing and finally the ending of the monthly menstrual periods. During and after menopause there are fewer female hormones circulating in the body, and women are more likely to gain weight, incur vaginal infections, high blood pressure, heart disease, and overt (recognised) diabetes. Emotional stress at this time in a woman's life may make diabetes harder to control.

MENSES, MENSTRUATION   In the female, it is the recurrent monthly discharge of blood and other substances that line the uterus (womb). For reasons not fully understood, menstruation may be irregular in the diabetic, and if so, and a pregnancy occurs, the date of delivery may be difficult to calculate. See also PREGNANCY AND CHILDBIRTH.

MENTAL STRESS   See STRESS.

MESSENGER RNA (mRNA)   See CELLS.

METABOLIC ACIDOSIS   An acid-base imbalance. Metabolic acidosis is a fall in the arterial blood or plasma pH to less than 7.35, and a fall in plasma total carbon dioxide (CO_2) content to less than 24 milliequivalents per litre, resulting in too much lactic acid and acetoacetic acid (a ketone body). The most common cause of metabolic acidosis is diabetic ketoacidosis (acidosis with high blood glucose and large amounts of ketones), but it is also seen in drug poisoning, especially with salicylates (the aspirin family), and in kidney failure. See also ACID-BASE BALANCE; DIABETIC KEOTACIDOSIS; HYPERGLYCAEMIC HYPEROSMOLAR NONKETOTIC COMA; LACTIC ACIDOSIS; pH SCALE.

METABOLIC ALKALOSIS   An acid-base imbalance. Metabolic alkalosis is a rise in the arterial blood or plasma pH to greater than 7.45, and a rise in plasma carbon dioxide (CO_2) content to greater than 30 milliequivalents per litre. Some symptoms of metabolic alkalosis are hypoventilation (under-breathing), irritability, and tetany (muscle spasms). Metabolic alkalosis can be caused by consuming too much alkali; for example, taking sodium bicarbonate (baking soda) for indigestion, especially when kidney disease is present. Other causes of metabolic alkalosis include loss of potassium with the use of diuretics (water pills), and loss of acid from the body, which can occur with prolonged vomiting. See also ACID-BASE BALANCE; pH SCALE.

METABOLISM   The two-part process in which foods are chemically changed in the body. In catabolism, food is broken down for use as energy at the cell level (also called respiration); in anabolism, body tissue is built up and repaired from food and other nutrients, a process also called synthesis. The process of metabolism is essential to life.

Insulin is the main anabolic hormone, keeping food from being wasted. See also BASAL METABOLIC RATE.

METER, METRE, M   See METRIC SYSTEM.

METHANOL   Methyl or wood alcohol. Poisonous. See ALCOHOL

METRIC SYSTEM   A system of measurement based on multiples of 10, as in our monetary system. With the exception of the United States and a few small countries, the entire world uses the metric system or is committed to it. Many large industries in the United States use the metric system, and pharmacists have been measuring in metrics for over twenty years. The popular 100-unit insulin and matching syringe is part of the change-over to the metric system.

Measurement in this country has consisted of several different systems. The avoirdupois system – 16 ounces in a pound – has been used for coarse weights. Fine measurements have been based on the apothecaries' system using the grain (gr) (originally the weights of a grain of wheat), and 12 ounces to the pound.

With three systems of measurement currently in operation, there is confusion – even resentment; however, we will soon become comfortable with the precision and simplicity of the metric system. Accurate measurement is imperative to anyone who takes drugs of any kind, and there must be no confusion in the changeover from grains (gr) to the grams (Gm, gm, g) of the metric system. Food will be weighed in grams and kilograms (kg); liquids in millitres (ml or mL), decilitres (dl), and litres (l); and linear measurements in millimetres (mm), centimetres (cm), metres (m), and kilometres (km). The Fahrenheit (F) temperature scale is being replaced by the Celsius (C) scale (formerly called centigrade), and conversion formulas are included in this section (see also THERMOMETER, CLINICAL).

The metre is the basic linear unit of the metric system: the unit of volume is the litre, and the unit of weight (mass), the gram. A $\frac{1}{100}$ of a metre is a *centimetre* (cm). A cube measuring 1 centimetre per side is a cubic centimetre (cc) and 1,000 cc is 1 litre (1). The gram is equal to the weight of 1 cc of pure water, 4°C, at sea level; therefore a litre of water weighs 1,000 grams, or 1 kilogram (kg). It was originally intended that a cube 1 decimetre (10 cm) on each side should be exactly the same as 1 litre, 1,000 cc; however, because of difficulty in measuring, a litre is 1.000028 cubic decimetres. By definition, ¹⁄₁₀₀₀ of a litre is 1 millilitre (ml), so a cc and an ml, although not exactly the same, are synonymous. They are used interchangeably, except in precise scientific measurements.

The decilitre (dl) is a term used more often today. It equals ¹⁄₁₀ of a litre, or 100 ml (cc). Laboratory terms previously expressed in 'mg %' or 'per 100 ml, or cc,' are now being shortened to 'per dl'. Examples of all three terms are: plasma glucose = 96 mg%; or 96 mg/100 ml or cc; or 96 mg/dl.

Metric Weight Measurement

1 gram	= 10 decigrams (dg)
„ „	= 100 centigrams (cg)
„ „	= 1,000 milligrams (mg)
„ „	= 1,000,000 micrograms (mcg or μg)
„ „	= 1,000,000,000 nanograms (ng)
10 grams	= 1 decagram (dkg)
100 grams	= 1 hectogram (hg)
1,000 grams	= 1 kilogram (kg)

Metric Linear Measure

1 metre	= 10 decimetres (dm)
„ „	= 100 centimetres (cm)
„ „	= 1,000 millimetres (mm)
„ „	= 1,000,000 micrometres (μm)
„ „	= 1,000,000,000 nanometres (nm)
10 metres	= 1 decametre (dkm)
100 metres	= 1 hectometre (hm)
1,000 metres	= 1 kilometre (km)
1 kilometre	= 0.6 miles

METRIC CONVERSION TABLES

A Partial List

WEIGHT (Mass)

When you know	You can find	If you multiply by
ounces	grams	28.
pounds	kilograms	0.45
milligrams	grams	0.001
grams	milligrams	1000.
kilograms	pounds	2.2

LIQUID (Volume)

When you know	You can find	If you multiply by
ounces	millilitres (cc)	30.
pints	litres	0.57
quarts	litres	1.14
gallons	litres	4.56
millilitres	ounces	0.034
decilitres	litres	10.
litres	pints	1.75
litres	quarts	0.88
litres	gallons	0.22

HOUSEHOLD MEASUREMENTS

1 teaspoon	4–5	millilitres (ml), or cubic centimetres (cc)
1 dessert spoon	10	millilitres
1 tablespoon	15	millilitres
¼ cup	60	millilitres
⅓ cup	80	millilitres
½ cup	120	millilitres
1 cup	240	millilitres
1 pint	600	millilitres
1 quart	1,200	millilitres
1 ounce (fluid)	30	millilitres

Temperature Equivalents

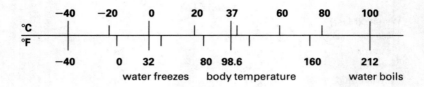

TEMPERATURE CONVERSION FORMULAS

$F = Fahrenheit \quad C = Celsius$

Fahrenheit to Celsius: The boiling point of water at sea level is 212°F.
To find the boiling point of water on the Celsius scale, use the formula
$C = 5/9 (F - 32)$:
$C = 5/9 (212 - 32)$
$C = 5/9 (180)$
$C = \dfrac{5 \times 180}{9}$
$C = \dfrac{900}{9}$
$C = 100°$
Celsius to Fahrenheit: The boiling point of water at sea level is 100°C.

To find the boiling point of water on the Fahrenheit scale, use the formula,
$F = (9/5 \times C) + 32$:
$F = (9/5 \times 100) + 32$
$F = \dfrac{9 \times 100}{5} + 32$
$F = \dfrac{900}{5} + 32$
$F = 180 + 32$
$F = 212°$

See THERMOMETER, CLINICAL. For further information on the metric system, write to the Metrication Board. See Directory.

MEXICAN-AMERICAN DIABETIC DIET See FOOD EX-CHANGES, Exchange List for Ethnic Foods.

174

MICROANGIOPATHY See BASEMENT CELLS MEMBRANE; BLOOD VESSEL DISEASE; KIDNEY DISEASE; RETINA, RETINOPATHY.

MICROANEURYSM See RETINA, RETINOPATHY.

MICROGRAM (mcg, μg) 1/1,000,000 of a gram. See METRIC SYSTEM.

MICRO-ORGANISMS Organisms too small to be seen by the naked eye. They possess characteristics and properties that are similar to plants and animals but are in a classification by themselves, called Protista. Some micro-organisms are pathogenic, capable of causing infection, serious disease, and death, whereas others are not harmful. Still others are beneficial to life; for example, the bacteria in the intestines help with the digestion of food and the manufacture of some vitamins.

The following is a classification of micro-organisms.

Bacteria are single-celled organisms. Streptococcus and Staphylococcus are bacteria.

Fungi exist as single- or multi-celled organisms, including the yeasts and moulds. Athlete's foot is caused by a fungus.

Viruses are obligate intracellular parasites, which means they must have a living animal, plant, or bacterium in which to grow, as they cannot reproduce by themselves. See also INFECTION AND INFLAMMATION; RESEARCH.

MICTURITION The act of urinating or voiding the bladder.

MIDSTREAM URINE SPECIMEN See URINE TESTS.

MIGRAINE HEADACHES See HEADACHES.

MILD-TYPE DIABETES This refers to diabetes that can be controlled by weight loss and diet. See also DIABETES MELLITUS, ADULT-ONSET.

MILK AND MILK POWDER See FOOD EXCHANGES, List 1.

MILK, HUMAN See PREGNANCY AND CHILDBIRTH.

MILLIGRAM (mg or mgm) $\frac{1}{1000}$ of a gram. See METRIC SYSTEM.

MILLILITRE (ml) $\frac{1}{1000}$ of a litre. The same as a cubic centimetre (cc) and used interchangeably. See METRIC SYSTEM.

MINERALOCORTICOIDS See ADRENAL GLANDS.

MINERALS Compounds that are inorganic – not coming

175

are calcium, phosphorus, potassium, sulphur, sodium, from living things. The major minerals needed by the body chlorine, and magnesium. Some other minerals needed by the body in smaller amounts, called 'trace' minerals, are iron, zinc, manganese, copper, and iodine. Chromium is associated with the utilisation of glucose in the body. See also CHROMIUM; NUTRIENTS.

MISCARRIAGE The ending of a pregnancy following the third month and before the seventh. See also PREGNANCY AND CHILDBIRTH.

MIXING BOTTLE or VIAL See INSULIN.

MODIFIED INSULIN Insulin that is changed by the addition of chemicals to prolong its action in the body. See also INSULIN.

MOLASSES See SUGAR.

MOLECULAR GENETICS See RESEARCH (Recombinant DNA).

MOLECULE The smallest amount of a substance that can exist in a free state and still retain its characteristics.

MONILIASIS See CANDIDA ALBICANS.

MONITORING OF BLOOD GLUCOSE (Blood Sugar) See RESEARCH.

MONOCYTE A white blood cell. See BLOOD.

MONOSACCHARIDES Simple sugars. See SUGAR.

MONOSODIUM GLUTAMATE (MSG) See SODIUM.

MONOUNSATURATED FATS The same as unsaturated fats. See LIPIDS.

MONTHLY PERIODS See MENSES, MENSTRUATION.

MORBIDITY A morbid or diseased state or condition. The morbidity rate is the amount of illness in a district, county, state, or country. See also DIABETES STATISTICS.

MORNING SICKNESS See PREGNANCY AND CHILDBIRTH.

MORTALITY RATE The number of people who die each year of a given disease compared with the total population.

MOTHER'S MILK See PREGNANCY AND CHILDBIRTH.

MOTION SICKNESS See TRAVELLING WITH DIABETES.

MOUTH CARE Good mouth care is important. Rough spots on the teeth or a poor bite can irritate the inside of the mouth and lead to infection. Diabetics do not seem to have more cavities than the average person, but those in poor control seem to have more abscessed teeth and problems with their gums. Dentists say the main reason for cavities is the excessive use of sugar in the Western world.

If you wear false teeth or partial plates, they must fit well to prevent sores. Sore gums that may bleed is gingivitis, and gums that produce pus is called pyorrhoea. See your dentist if these problems occur, and keep follow-up appointments. See also CANDIDA ALBICANS.

MSG See SODIUM.

MUCOSA, MUCOUS MEMBRANE Tissue that lines the passages and cavities of the digestive, respiratory, and genitourinary tracts. See also DIGESTION.

MUMPS Mumps is a virus disease (see MICRO-ORGANISMS) primarily affecting the parotid glands, the glands that make saliva; it is also called epidemic parotitis. Mumps can cause damage to ovaries in the female and testes in the male, and there is some evidence that mumps virus may also damage pancreatic cells, causing diabetes. See also RESEARCH.

MUSCLE BIOPSY See BIOPSY.

MUSCLE SPASMS See tetany under METABOLIC ALKALOSIS.

MUSCLE WASTING See INTEROSSEOUS WASTING.

MYELIN SHEATH See NERVOUS SYSTEM.

MYOCARDIAL INFARCTION (MI) A heart attack in which there is damage to the heart muscle. See also DIABETES STATISTICS; HEART DISEASE.

MYOCARDIUM See HEART DISEASE.

N

NAILS See FEET, CARE OF; HANDS.

NARCOTIC This includes opium, opium derivatives, and other powerful pain-killing drugs that produce stupor or sleep. Strictly speaking, a drug that induces sleep but is not a pain killer is a hypnotic. Narcotics and hypnotics are habit-forming and must be prescribed by a physician. Do not take more than the recommended dose, and do not borrow from friends. The diabetic person should be especially careful to avoid substances, such as narcotics, that can mask diabetic symptoms or provide a sense of unreality, since this can interfere with the control of diabetes.

NAUSEA Nausea is a sick feeling in the stomach and may or may not be followed by vomiting. Nausea may indicate low blood glucose. Prolonged vomiting, especially accompanied by diarrhoea, may cause dehydration and loss of potassium. Do not treat this lightly because it may mean a viral or bacterial infection is present; in any case it means little or no food is being digested, which can lead to hypoglycaemic reactions. Call your doctor. See also HYPOGLYCAEMIC REACTIONS; TRAVELLING WITH DIABETES.

NECROBIOSIS LIPOIDICA DIABETICORUM See SKIN DISEASES.

NECROTIC TISSUE Dead tissue.

NEEDLES See INSULIN SYRINGES AND THEIR CARE.

NEGATIVE TEST A laboratory test that produces no reaction, meaning a normal reaction or a reaction within normal ranges. The opposite is a positive test, which indicates a reaction outside the normal ranges. See also BLOOD TESTS; URINE TESTS.

NEONATE A newborn infant, up to the first four weeks after birth. See PREGNANCY AND CHILDBIRTH.

NEOVASCULARISATION The development of new blood vessels, especially on the retina, after the original blood vessels become clogged or ruptured. See also RETINA, RETINOPATHY.

NEPHRITIS Bright's Disease – inflammation of the kidney. See also KIDNEY DISEASE.

NEPHRON The functional unit of the kidneys. See KID-NEYS.

NEPHROPATHY Kidney disease.

NEPHROSIS Degenerative changes in the kidney. See KID-NEY DISEASE.

NEPHROTIC SYNDROME Kidney disease of any kind.

NERVE DEAFNESS Loss of hearing as a result of damage to the nerves serving the ear. It is rare as a complication of diabetes. See also DIABETIC NEUROPATHY.

NERVOUS SYSTEM The entire nervous system is interconnected, but for purposes of description it is divided into two parts: the central nervous system, which includes the brain and the spinal cord, and the peripheral nervous system, which includes the cranial and spinal nerves and the autonomic nervous sytem. The cranial nerves issue from the lower brain and brain stem in twelve pairs; they serve the face, eyes, ears, nose, tongue, neck, shoulders, throat, lungs, heart, stomach, gall bladder, and intestines. The spinal nerves have thirty-one pairs of nerves branching off the spinal cord and connect with the autonomic nervous system. The autonomic nervous system is an 'automatic' nervous system having two parts: the sympathetic and the parasympathetic systems. The autonomic system controls the activities of the body that we do not think about, such as the functioning of the heart. It makes the blood vessels tight and small, or relaxed and large, varying the supply of blood to different parts of the body as needed. It controls the movements in the digestive tract and the glands and their secretions. The two divisions of the autonomic nervous system, the sympathetic and the parasympathetic, work together in a complicated manner to turn things off and on in the body. Disease of the nervous system can affect any part of the body.

Many nerve fibres are covered with a fatty white material known as the myelin sheath. Continuous high levels of blood glucose may cause this protective covering to disintegrate, causing nerve damage. See also DIABETIC NEUROPATHY.

NEUROGENIC BLADDER   See URINARY BLADDER.

NEUROGLYCOPOENIA   A condition in which the blood glucose is so low that too little glucose reaches the nerves, and specifically the brain. The symptoms may be lack of concentration, irritability, and other changes in behaviour. When glucose is not available, ketone bodies can be used to provide energy and nourishment to the brain. See also KETONE BODIES.

NEUROLOGY   The study of diseases of the nervous system. A medical specialist who treats these diseases is called a neurologist.

NEUROPATHY   See DIABETIC NEUROPATHY.

NEUTRAL FATS   See LIPIDS.

NEUTRAL PROTAMINE HAGEDORN INSULIN   NPH insulin. See INSULIN.

NEUTROPHIL   A white blood cell. See BLOOD.

NIACIN, or NICOTINIC ACID   Part of the vitamin B complex. Niacin may cause temporary hot flushes or a warmth or flushing in the face. A form of niacin, nicotinamide, does not cause flushing. Niacin in large doses is used to lower blood cholesterol; however, it must be taken only under a doctor's orders because it can raise the blood glucose. Niacin is found normally in meat, fish, poultry, eggs, vegetables, fruit, cereal grains, and rice.

NITROGEN BALANCE   Nitrogen enters the body when protein is eaten. A healthy person eats about the same amount of nitrogen as he loses. When the body loses more protein than is eaten, the result is a negative nitrogen balance. Disease, such as kidney disease, can also cause negative nitrogen balance. An excess of protein results in a positive nitrogen balance. Extra protein is needed during growth and pregnancy, for recovery from certain diseases, and to promote healing.

NOCTURIA   See ENURESIS.

NONACIDOTIC DIABETES   See DIABETES MELLITUS, ADULT-ONSET.

NONCALORIC   Containing no calories.

NONKETOTIC DIABETES See DIABETES MELLITUS, ADULT-ONSET.

NONKETOTIC HYPEROSMOLAR COMA See HYPER-GLYCAEMIC HYPEROSMOLAR NONKETOTIC COMA.

NONPRESCRIPTION DRUGS Medication bought over the counter (OTC drugs) without a doctor's prescription. Many drugs interact with others, either lessening their effect or enhancing it. Vitamin C in doses of 1,000 milligrams (1 gram) can change the results of a urine test, and ordinary aspirin can interact with oral hypoglycaemic agents, producing low blood glucose. These are only two examples. *Taking any drugs without consulting your doctor can be dangerous!* See also SALICYLATES; URINE TESTS.

NONPYROGENIC Sterile; noninfectious.

NONTOXIC Not poisonous.

NORMAL SALINE A solution of sodium chloride similar in salt content to the blood. Used at times to dilute insulin when insulin is given in very small doses. See INSULIN.

NORMOGLYCAEMIA A normal amount of glucose in the blood.

NOSEBLEED The medical name is epistaxis. The most common causes of nosebleed are nose-picking, blowing the nose hard and frequently, and high blood pressure. Treatment: Tilt the head back and sit quietly with a wet, cold towel over the nose, and one at the back of the neck. Do not breathe through or blow the nose during this time. If the bleeding does not stop in a few minutes, gently pack the nostril with gauze. If the bleeding does not stop in 15 to 20 minutes, or if it is profuse, call your doctor or go to the nearest hosptial. A serious nosebleed can be stressful, and the reason for the bleeding should be treated, especially if it is a recurring problem.

NPH INSULIN An intermediate-acting insulin. See also INSULIN.

NPO In preparation for surgery or certain tests, it means 'nothing per os' or nothing by mouth; however, sometimes you may drink water, so be sure to ask. Always drink water before an oral glucose tolerance test (see under BLOOD TESTS) because you will be asked to produce urine specimens several times during the test.

NUCLEIC ACIDS; NUCLEUS   See CELLS.

NUCLEOTIDE   The basic structural unit of nucleic acids. See also CELLS.

NUMBNESS   See PARAESTHESIA.

NURSES   A state registered nurse (SRN) has undergone 3 years of training; a state enrolled nurse (SEN) 2 years. District nurses (D/N) who visit patients in their homes to assist with injections, dressings and general care, are usually SRNs. Health visitors are also SRNs but have undergone additional training and advise about such matters as home conditions. Some doctors have attached to their surgery a community liaison nurse who is specially trained in diabetes.

NURSES   If needed, nurses can be hired to travel with you. See TRAVELLING WITH DIABETES.

NURSING MOTHER   See PREGNANCY AND CHILDBIRTH.

NUTRIENTS   Food, vitamins, and minerals needed by the body to make tissue for growth and replacement and to give energy and heat. See also METABOLISM.

NUTRITION   The use and study of food and how food is utilised in the body. Persons engaged in this work are dietitians and nutritionists. There is no degree given in nutrition, but many nutritionists are medical doctors, biochemists, and other people with advanced degrees who have furthered their studies in the area of food and nutrition. See also REGISTERED DIETITIAN.

NUTRITIONAL OEDEMA   See OEDEMA.

NUTRITION LABELLING   Any food to which a nutrient has been added or for which a nutrition claim is made must, by law, carry a nutrition statement on its label.

NUTRITIVE SWEETENERS   See SUGAR.

NUTS   See FOOD EXCHANGES, List 6.

O

OBESITY See WEIGHT.

OCCLUDE To shut or stop up; to close, or clog.

OCEAN TRAVEL See TRAVELLING WITH DIABETES.

OCULAR Concerning the eyes. See EYESIGHT.

OCULIST See OPHTHALMOLOGIST.

OEDEMA The common name for oedema is dropsy; it is an excessive accumulation of water in the tissues that is sometimes present in heart and kidney disease. It is also called fluid retention. In testing a person for oedema, the doctor pushes against the skin over the shins and around the feet and ankles. If excess water is present in the body, applying pressure to the skin will make pits that remain for a while; this is called 'pitting oedema'. With a stethoscope, excess fluid in the lungs is heard as 'rales', a frying type of sound. Another symptom is puffiness of the fingers and around the eyes. Fluid is held in the body tissues when the kidneys fail to rid the body of excess sodium, or the heart fails to pump properly. See also HEART DISEASE; SODIUM.

Nutritional oedema A condition in which extra fluid is present in the tissues because the person has not eaten enough protein, or enough complete protein (protein containing all the essential amino acids). See AMINO ACIDS.

OESOPHAGUS The gullet; part of the alimentary canal starting at the back of the mouth and leading to the stomach. See also INDIGESTION.

OGTT, or GTT Oral Glucose Tolerance Test. See BLOOD TESTS.

OIL See LIPIDS.

OLIGURIA A very small output of urine. Present in dehydration and in advance kidney disease. See also KIDNEY DISEASE.

ONE-DROP CLINITEST See URINE TESTS.

OPHTHALMOLOGIST A medical specialist who treats diseases and disorders of the eye. Also called an oculist. See also EYESIGHT.

OPHTHALMOSCOPE An instrument for examining the interior of the eye, consisting mainly of a mirror that reflects a light through the pupil of the eye. The retina, or back of the eye, can be inspected with this instrument.

OPTICIAN One who grinds, fits, adjusts, and sells the eyeglasses prescribed by the ophthalmologist or optometrist.

ORAL CONTRACEPTIVES See CONTRACEPTIVES.

ORAL DIABETIC AGENTS See ORAL HYPOGLYCAEMIC AGENTS.

ORAL GLUCOSE TOLERANCE TEST (OGTT, or GTT) See BLOOD TESTS.

ORAL HYPOGLYCAEMIC AGENTS (OHAs) 90 to 95 per cent of diabetics have adult-onset diabetes. (see DIABETES MELLITUS, ADULT-ONSET), and about 80 per cent of these can be treated by diet, weight reduction, and exercise. When patients fail to follow this regimen or refuse to use insulin, oral hypoglycaemic agents in the form of pills can be used to lower the blood glucose. These agents are not oral insulin (insulin taken by mouth is destroyed by the digestive juices in the stomach), but are sulphonylureas, which are related to the sulpha drugs (see SULPHONAMIDES). Sulphonylureas must not be taken by the person who has a known allergy to the sulphas.

The University Group Diabetes Program (UGDP) was a study by a group of university scientists in 1959 designed to evaluate the long-term effects of tolbutamide (Orinase) and insulin in reducing the complications of blood vessel disease in patients receiving these medications. Some patients received regular tolbutamide pills and some were given fake pills called placebos, although they were not told this. In 1962 phenformin was added to the study. Tolbutamide was dropped from the study in 1969, because it was felt there was an increased death rate among those patients receiving it as compared with the placebo group and insulin-treated groups. In 1971 phenformin was discontinued for similar reasons. The completed report states that there is doubt as to the effectiveness of *any* hypoglycaemic agent, including insulin, in controlling or preventing blood vessel disease. This report has been challenged by many diabetologists and statisticians, because it was felt that the research was not planned on a sound scientific basis, and further research is needed.

Two types of OHAs have been in use until recently: the solphonylureas, already mentioned, and the biguanides. The use of biguanides, however, has been limited because of the danger of lactic acidosis.

There are seven sulphonylureas used widely in the United Kingdom. Each acts in generally the same way to lower the blood glucose by stimulating the beta cells of the pancreas to release insulin and to inhibit the release of glucose from the liver. The main difference among the seven types is in the duration of action. Sulphonylureas are definitely not useful for the diabetic who does not produce any insulin; and patients who take an oral hypoglycaemic agent may require treatment with insulin during periods of mental and physical stress, such as illness, infection, surgery, or pregnancy and childbirth. Usually insulin can be discontinued after the period of stress is over and treatment with OHAs resumed. The choice regarding which oral agent a patient should use must be up to the doctor, who will judge each patient individually. His instructions should be followed closely; if you do not understand the instructions initially, ask him again until you do understand them, because in the wrong doses these drugs can cause the blood glucose to become too low. None of the oral agents should be used when significant liver or kidney disease is present.

GENERAL INSTRUCTIONS: Never omit meals. If you become sick, take urine tests for sugar and acetone, take your temperature, and call the doctor.

Hypoglycaemic Reactions   Low blood glucose usually has a slower onset with OHAs than with insulin. It may creep up rather insidiously, with a feeling of fatigue, or malaise. Second-voided urine tests will be negative. If eating some glucose is not helpful, be sure to let your doctor know what is happening. If you have lost a large amount of weight without a reduction of dosage of your pills, the doctor may want to evaluate this. Taking alcohol in combination with the OHAs may cause a flushing of the face (Antabuse-like reactions – see ALCOHOL).

185

Drug Interactions When other drugs are taken in combination with oral hypoglycaemic agents, low blood glucose may occur in some cases. Those most noted for this effect are alcohol (with Orinase and Diabinese), aspirin and other salicylates in large doses, sulpha drugs, anabolic steroids, chloramphenicol, Tanderil, nicotinic acid, Atromid-S, Butazolidin, and Benemid.

WARNING: Keep these drugs out of the reach of children! Should a child ingest them accidentally, try to determine how many were swallowed, and the name and strength of the pill. This is a medical emergency. If you cannot talk to a doctor on the phone for instructions, take the child to the nearest hospital.

Oral Hypoglycaemic Agents – Sulphonylureas See table on page 187.

ORAL INSULIN There is no such thing as oral insulin at this time. Insulin is destroyed by the digestive juices of the stomach. See also ORAL HYPOGLYCAEMIC AGENTS; RESEARCH.

ORANGE JUICE For low blood glucose, give ½ cup without added sugar. See FOOD EXCHANGES, List 3; HYPOGLYCAEMIC REACTIONS.

ORGANIC Living things, or composed of living things, such as plants or animals.

ORGAN MEATS Brain, kidneys, liver, pancreas, and thymus. Rich in vitamin B complex. Liver is high in vitamin A, and liver and brains are high in cholesterol. See also FOOD EXCHANGES, List 5 (Medium-Fat Meat).

ORIENTAL DIABETIC DIET See FOOD EXCHANGES, Exchange Lists for Ethnic Foods.

ORINASE See ORAL HYPOGLYCAEMIC AGENTS.

ORTHOPAEDIC SURGEON A medical doctor who specialises in the prevention or correction of deformities and diseases of the limbs, bones, muscles, joints, and other parts relating to movement.

ORTHOSTATIC HYPOTENSION See BLOOD PRESSURE.

OSMOSIS, OSMOTIC DIURESIS Osmosis is a natural event in which a solvent, such as water, passes through a cell membrane, from a solution that is dilute into a solution that is more concentrated. For example, fresh water is

ORAL HYPOGLYCAEMIC AGENTS – SULPHONYLUREAS

CHEMICAL OR GENERIC NAME	TRADE NAME	TABLETS	DOSE	PEAK EFFECT	DURATION OF ACTION	SIDE EFFECTS
ACETOHEXAMIDE	DIMELOR	Yellow Round 500 mg	250-1,500 mg/d	8-12 hours	12-24 hours	Uncommon
CHLORPROPAMIDE	DIABINESE	White Round 100 or 250 mg	100-500 mg/d	6-18 hours	up to 36 hours	Low blood glucose at night in old people
GLIBENGLAMIDE	EUGLUCON DAONIL	White *Oblong* (5 mg) White *Round* (2.5 mg)	2.5-30 mg/d	4-8 hours	up to 15 hours	Low blood glucose if initial dose too high
GLIPIZIDE	GLIBENESE	White Oblong 5 mg	2.5-30 mg/d	6-8 hours	8-12 hours	May interact with other drugs
GLYMIDINE	GONDAFON	White Oblong 500 mg	500-1,000 mg/d	?	up to 24 hours	Uncommon
TOLAZAMIDE	TOLANASE	White Round 100 or 250 mg	100-1,000 mg/d	6-8 hours	up to 12 hours	Uncommon
TOLBUTAMIDE	RASTINON ORINASE	White Round 500 mg	500-3,000 mg/d	4-8 hours	6-12 hours	Rashes ⎫ Rare Anaemia ⎭

always drawn into cells existing in salt water (brine). Osmotic pressure is the ability of a solution to draw water from another solution across a cell membrane, eventually equalising the concentration of both. Osmolality is the strength or osmotic effectiveness of the solution, and is written as milliosmoles/kilogram of solvent. Osmolarity is the number of osmotically active particles per litre of solution; for example, plasma. Hyperosmolality is the abnormal concentration of solutes in the blood, such as glucose or electrolytes. Osmotic diuresis occurs when the blood glucose is high, as in diabetic ketoacidosis or hyperglycaemic hyperosmolar nonketotic coma; the glucose exerts osmotic pressure, drawing water from the cells and from extracellular (interstitial) spaces into the blood. This extra volume of fluid is excreted in the urine along with glucose, causing great thirst and dangerous dehydration throughout the body. Electrolyte imbalance also occurs at this time. See also ELECTROLYTES.

OUNCE From the apothecaries' measure (see). See also METRIC SYSTEM.

OUTPATIENT A patient given care at a hospital without being admitted. Such day care can include access to clinics, the emergency room, minor surgery, X-rays, and laboratories.

OVERDOSE See DRUG OVERDOSE.

OVERNIGHT FAST See FASTING; NPO.

OVERT DIABETES Diabetes that has symptoms leading to a positive diagnosis. See also Classification of Diabetes under DIABETES MELLITUS.

OVER-THE-COUNTER DRUGS (OTC) See NONPRESCRIPTION DRUGS.

OVERWEIGHT See WEIGHT.

OXYGEN One of the chemical element gases in the air we breathe, and necessary to life.

OXYTOCIN See PREGNANCY AND CHILDBIRTH.

P

PACKED CELL VOLUME (PCV) Also called **Haema-tocrit**. See BLOOD TESTS.

PAIN A feeling of distress. There are two general types of pain: acute, having a rapid onset and short course; and chronic, having a long duration. Hyperaesthesia is a term for pain, used when it is caused by nerve damage. See also DIABETIC NEUROPATHY; LEG PAIN.

PALENESS Pallor. If your face becomes pale suddenly, your blood glucose may be low. See HYPOGLYCAEMIC REACTIONS.

PALLIATIVE A treatment or drug that eases medical problems but does not cure anything. Pain pills are an example; the pill takes away or dulls the pain, but it does not treat the reason for the pain.

PALPITATION A 'fluttering' heartbeat. The affected individual is usually aware that his heart is beating irregularly. This could happen to anyone, and often does, and usually disappears as fast as it comes; however, it could signify low blood glucose. If you experience any change in your heart rate or rhythm, especially if chest and arm pain (left arm, right arm, or both) accompanies it, call your doctor immediately, as it may be the signal of more serious heart problems. See also HEART DISEASE.

PANADOL See PARACETAMOL. See also SALICYLATES.

PANCREAS A gland about 6 by 1½ inches located behind the lower portion of the stomach. The pancreas is both an endocrine and an exocrine gland. The endocrine functions are associated with a group of cells called the islets of Langerhans. These islet cells are of at least three kinds: alpha, beta, and delta cells. The alpha cells produce glucagon; beta cells produce insulin; and delta cells produce a somatostatin-like material. The exocrine parts excrete large amounts of alkaline digestive juices (1,500-3,000 cc's/day) that neutralise stomach acids as food enters the small intestine and also furnish enzymes for digestion.

189

Pancreatitis   An inflammation of the pancreas caused by gall bladder disease, damage by viruses such as mumps, and alcoholism. There is severe abdominal pain in the upper abdomen, radiating to the side and back, usually lasting for several days. Nausea may be present, with back pain, lack of appetite, and an increase in body temperature. The patient is usually sick enough to require hospitalisation. Chronic pancreatitis over a period of 10 to 20 years is often accompanied by diarrhoea. Damage to islet cells can cause a transient increase in blood glucose by decreasing the production of insulin, and may permanently damage these cells, causing diabetes.

Pancreatic Carcinoma   An insidious form of cancer because it is so difficult to detect; however, there is a new technique of scanning the pancreas and other organs, called ultrasonography, that can detect abnormal masses or tumours much earlier than was previously possible. Angiography can be performed as a follow-up to ultrasonography to determine if lifesaving surgery is practical.

PANCREATIC IMPLANTS   See RESEARCH.

PARACETAMOL   A pain killer sold as Panadol. It is suitable for diabetics.

PARAESTHESIA   Prickling, or loss of sensation occurring mostly in the feet and hands and caused more often by nerve disease than by blood vessel disease. This feeling loss is sometimes called the 'glove and stocking effect'. Another term is Hypoaesthesia, meaning a decrease in sensation or feeling. Control of diabetes by lowering blood glucose levels to normal levels often helps with these problems. See also DIABETIC NEUROPATHY.

PARALYTIC BLADDER   See URINARY BLADDER.

PARASYMPATHETIC NERVOUS SYSTEM   See NERVOUS SYSTEM.

PARENTERAL INJECTION   Injection of medication through the skin. See also INSULIN INJECTION AND INJECTION SITES.

PARTIAL PLATES   See MOUTH CARE.

PASS THROUGH OF COLOURS   See URINE TESTS.

PATHOGEN   Any disease-producing agent or micro-organism. See also MICRO-ORGANISMS.

PATHOLOGICAL Also **Pathogenic**. Refers to pathology, the study of the nature and cause of disease. Pathogens are micro-organisms capable of causing disease. See also INFECTION AND INFLAMMATION; MICRO-ORGANISMS.

-PATHY A word ending meaning 'disease of', or an abnormal condition; for example, nephropathy is kidney disease (a nephron is a basic part of the kidney).

PEAK OF ACTION The time at which drug dosage is most effective.

PAEDIATRICIAN A medical doctor especially trained to care for the diseases of children.

PENIS See GENITALIA.

PERIDONTAL DISEASE Disease of the gums. See also MOUTH CARE.

PERIPHERAL Referring to the edges or outside.

PERIPHERAL NERVOUS SYSTEM See NERVOUS SYSTEM.

PERIPHERAL VASCULAR DISEASE Disease related to lack of a good blood supply to the legs and feet. See also BLOOD VESSEL DISEASE; LEG PAIN.

PERIPHERAL VISION See BLINDNESS.

PERITONEAL DIALYSIS See KIDNEY DISEASE.

PERSPIRATION See SWEATING.

pH See pH SCALE.

PHACO-EMULSIFICATION (PE) See EYESIGHT.

PHAEOCHROMOCYTOMA See ADRENAL GLANDS; TUMOURS.

PHARMACEUTICAL Referring to drugs and medicines, or to a pharmacy or drug business.

PHARMACIST A druggist; a person licensed to prepare and dispense medicines. The license is granted after a four-year college course of study, and in some states, an internship in a pharmacy. A pharmacist cannot prescribe medication, which is the function solely of a doctor.

PhD Doctor of Philosophy. A degree conferred by a college or university in a given department of knowledge. This degree is often necessary in order that the person may teach or conduct research.

PHENFORMIN HC1 (Hydrochloride) See ORAL HYPO-GLYCAEMIC AGENTS.

PHLEBITIS   Inflammation of a vein.

PHLEBOTOMY   See VENAPUNCTURE.

PHOSPHOLIPIDS   See LIPIDS.

PHOTOCOAGULATION   See RETINA, RETINOPATHY.

PHOTOSENSITIVITY   A condition in which the skin is extra sensitive to sunlight, and therefore more likely to burn. Various drugs may produce increased sensitivity to the sun, including oral hypoglycaemic agents, some diuretics (water pills), tranquillisers, and antibiotics. If you are taking any of these, check with your doctor or pharmacist about the possibility of photosensitivity; if it exists avoid overexposure to the sun.

pH SCALE   pH is the chemical symbol representing a scale that measures acidity vs alkalinity. A neutral solution, such as pure water, is said to have a pH of 7; anything below 7 is acid (vinegar is 2.3), and anything above 7 is alkaline (lye is 13). The scale runs from 0.00, total acidity, to 14, total alkalinity. pH actually represents the hydrogen (H) ion concentration of a solution; 'p' stands for the power of the hydrogen ion. The progression from one number to the next is tenfold; for example, a pH of 8 is ten times greater than a pH of 7.

   The normal pH of blood is 7.35 to 7.45; this means that blood is slightly alkaline. The normal pH of urine ranges from 4.8 to 8.0, which means that urine can be acid or alkaline.

   The tests for blood or urine pH do not require food or drink restrictions prior to testing, unless the doctor gives special instructions. See also ACIDOSIS; ALKALOSIS; Ions under ELECTROLYTES.

PHYSICAL ACTIVITY   See EXERCISE/SPORTS (includes a diet for exercise); MANUAL LABOUR.

PHYSICAL STRESS   See STRESS.

PHYSICIAN   A medical doctor (MD), licensed and authorised by law to treat diseases.

PHYSIOLOGY   The study dealing with the function of various parts and organs of living organisms. An individual specialising in this science is called a physiologist.

PINT   See METRIC SYSTEM.

PIPE SMOKING   See discussion of smoking under TOBACCO.

PITUITARY GLAND (Hypophysis)   An endocrine gland. Sometimes called the master gland of the body, because it regulates growth, reproduction, and body metabolism. It is a small gland located in a small bony cavity beneath the base of the brain. See also DIABETES INSIPIDUS; GLANDS.

PITUITARY ABLATION   See RETINA, RETINOPATHY.

PLACEBO, PLACEBO EFFECT   The so-called sugar pill or capsule. This type of pill usually consists of milk sugar (lactose) and is used mainly in research. 'Placebo effect' is a term used when the person given a placebo without his knowledge is observed to be affected or claims to be affected by it in some way.

PLACENTA   A structure attached to the inside of the uterus (womb), which grows along with the unborn baby, and is attached to the baby by the umbilical cord. Through a system of exchange in the placenta, the baby gets its food and other substances from the blood of the mother. See also PREGNANCY AND CHILDBIRTH.

PLAIN INSULIN   Soluble insulin.   See INSULIN.

PLANE TRIPS.   See TRAVELLING WITH DIABETES.

PLAQUE   See HEART DISEASE.

PLASMA   See BLOOD.

PLASMA GLUCOSE   See GLUCOSE.

PLASMA INSULIN LEVELS   See BLOOD TESTS.

PLASTIC SYRINGES   See INSULIN SYRINGES AND THEIR CARE.

PLATELETS (Thrombocytes)   See BLOOD; Platelet Count under BLOOD TESTS; RESEARCH.

PLATES   Dentures. See MOUTH CARE.

PNEUMATURIA   See URINE.

POISON   See DRUG OVERDOSE; FOOD POISONING; SICKNESS.

POLYDIPSIA   An abnormal thirst. It is a symptom of diabetes insipidus, and uncontrolled diabetes mellitus. Polydipsia is accompanied by polyuria.

POLYHYDRAMNIOS   Excess amniotic fluid. See PLACENTA; PREGNANCY AND CHILDBIRTH; TOXAEMIA OF PREGNANCY.

POLYNEUROPATHY Disease of many nerves. See DIA-
BETIC NEUROPATHY; NERVOUS SYSTEM.

POLYOL PATHWAY Polyols are sugar alcohols. See cataracts under EYESIGHT; RESEARCH; SUGAR.

POLYPHAGIA Hunger and overeating. Despite eating more
food, weight loss may occur. This is especially true in
juvenile-onset diabetes, and may be one of the first symptoms. See DIABETES MELLITUS, JUVENILE-ONSET.

POLYSACCHARIDES Polysaccharides, complex sugars,
literally means 'many sugars', and refers to the starches.
Cellulose is a polysaccharide that humans cannot digest.
Inulin is a polysaccharide found in Jerusalem and globe
artichokes, onions and garlic. It is poorly absorbed from the
intestinal tract and so has little significance in terms of
calories, although when inulin is stored, the starch breaks
down to sugar. It is not known how long a period of storage
effects this change. Bananas, as they turn yellow with
brown spots, become less starchy and increase in sugar
content. In animals, glycogen, a polysaccharide, is stored in
the muscles and liver as an available source of glucose. See
also GLYCOGEN; STARCHES; SUGAR.

POLYUNSATURATED FATS AND OILS See LIPIDS

POLYURIA An abnormal production of urine. See also
POLYDIPSIA.

POOR CIRCULATION See BLOOD; HEART DISEASE;
LEG PAIN.

POP See SOFT DRINKS.

PORCINE, or PORK, INSULIN Insulin prepared from the
pancreas of pigs. See INSULIN.

POSITIVE TEST See NEGATIVE TEST.

POSTPRANDIAL Prandial refers to a meal, and postprandial means after a meal. See also Two-Hour Postprandial
Test under BLOOD TESTS.

POSTURAL HYPOTENSION See BLOOD PRESSURE.

POTASSIUM (K) A chemical element; one of the electrolytes
in the tissues and cells of the body. Potassium is present in
every cell of the body and is necessary to life. When it is lost
from the body through the use of diuretics (water pills) or by
prolonged vomiting, diarrhoea, or excessive sweating,
serious electrolyte imbalance may occur. When potassium is

lost the blood glucose rises. Bananas are a rich source of potassium. See also BLOOD TESTS; ELECTROLYTES.

POTATOES See FOOD EXCHANGES, List 4.

POTENTIATION The ability of one drug to enhance the action of another. Be sure your doctor knows all the medication you are taking, including nonprescription (over-the-counter) drugs.

POULTRY See FOOD EXCHANGES, List 5 (Lean Meat).

POUND Avoirdupois measurement. See METRIC SYSTEM.

PRECURSOR OF INSULIN See INSULIN.

PREDIABETIC See Classification of Diabetes under DIABETES MELLITUS.

PRE-ECLAMPSIA See PREGNANCY AND CHILDBIRTH.

PREGNANCY AND CHILDBIRTH Approximately one out of one hundred pregnant women are known diabetics. Before the availability of insulin, however, few diabetic women conceived or carried a pregnancy to term. Today, with strict control of blood glucose and newly available tests to evaluate the health of the mother and foetus, most women with diabetes can bear healthy children. Pregnancy is stressful to all women and to the diabetic in particular because the body produces more blood in pregnancy and increases the production of hormones – progesterone, oestrogen, and lactogen. These hormones all work against insulin; thus, pregnancy is described as being a diabetogenic state or condition, and each succeeding pregnancy is increasingly diabetogenic – it tends to cause diabetes in women who are genetically prone to it. It has been shown that about one out of one hundred pregnant women develop gestational diabetes, or diabetes caused by the stress of pregnancy. After delivery, most of these women have normal blood glucose in 4 to 6 weeks; however, half become overt diabetics within 15 years.

Only a short time ago women with diabetes were often advised to avoid pregnancy. But since the desire to bear a child is very strong in many women, most doctors today will counsel a woman carefully, so that she and her husband may make a wise decision. (The heredity of diabetes is greatly disputed today; see HEREDITY). Other important factors affecting this decision are the age of the mother, how long she has had diabetes, and how severe her diabetes is. If retinopathy and kidney disease are already present, they may worsen with pregnancy, and heart disease may also rule out childbearing.

Management of diabetes during pregnancy demands the very best of medical care. From beginning to end the prospective mother will visit the doctor more frequently than average, and will be subjected to a strict regimen including diet, insulin dosage, if needed, and many tests. Oral hypoglycaemic agents cannot be used during pregnancy because, unlike insulin, they cross the placental barrier, and may cause congenital defects in the infant. Those who cannot be controlled by diet will be placed on insulin, at least during the pregnancy.

Pregnancy is divided into three time periods, called trimesters: from conception through week 13: week 14 through week 27; and week 28 through week 40, a total of 240 days, when the average delivery or confinement takes place. The first trimester is the time when the mother may have what is commonly known as morning sickness – nausea and possibly vomiting. This can complicate diabetic control, and the doctor should be consulted as to the best way to handle each individual case. It is also during the first trimester that insulin dosage will probably be decreased because at that time metabolism is increased and there is a greater sensitivity to insulin. In the second and third trimesters, the need for insulin commonly increases until about the 36th week. The usual pattern for insulin is to give ⅔ of the total daily dose in the morning and ⅓ in the evening before supper, using a mixture of an intermediate acting insulin and regular insulin. See METABOLISM.

Diet in Pregnancy The diet must be adjusted to meet the needs of the mother and the developing infant. A pregnant diabetic woman who has normal weight is often encouraged to increase her caloric intake by 200 – 500 calories over her pre-pregnancy level. The mother will need an increase of 200 – 500 calories per day, mostly in carbohydrate, to help prevent ketosis. It is important to spread the caloric intake over the entire day. This may be done by dividing the total calories into 9 parts and distributing them as follows: ⅔ for breakfast, lunch and supper each, and ⅕ each at midmorning, midafternoon, and bedtime snacks. Smoking is not recommended during pregnancy.

Tests During Pregnancy   These include strict attention to urine testing; the doctor will usually advise using the two-drop Clinitest because it is more sensitive. If the test shows 1 per cent or more glucose, check for acetone and contact the doctor if the acetone test is positive. Many doctors are suggesting the use of Dextrostix because it allows a closer check on blood glucose. (For tests for nursing mothers, see Lactation at the end of this section). The aim is to maintain the blood glucose as close as possible, avoiding hypoglycaemia. A rise in blood pressure and an abnormal weight gain forecast the possibility of toxaemia of pregnancy, which is more prevalent in the mother with diabetes. If the prospective mother is threatened by toxaemia, she will be hospitalised for treatment to prevent harm to the foetus, or possible spontaneous abortion. The doctor will monitor the foetal heartbeat, and may perform amniocentesis. This is done by inserting a needlelike instrument through the abdominal wall and withdrawing a sample of amniotic fluid for tests. A decrease in phospholipids called lecithin/sphingomyelin, or an L/S ratio below 3.5, carries a risk of respiratory distress syndrome. Other tests can be made to evaluate placental function and foetal health by measuring hormones in the urine and blood. Ultrasonography is used to visualise the size and placement of the placenta, the amount of amniotic fluid, and the size and development of the foetus.

There is a risk of three to four times the normal number of foetal deaths and twice as many birth defects in the baby of the diabetic mother. The baby is always considered to be a high-risk baby who will need extra care and attention after birth. If the doctor does not suggest it, the parents should ask that a paediatrician stand by to care for the baby after delivery. The baby may be thin, but poorly controlled diabetics, and especially latent diabetics, are well known for producing fat babies, puffy from excess water, weighing 9 pounds or more. The size of the baby can be controlled to some extent by strict control of the blood glucose. Since glucose passes through the placenta to the baby (foetus), the

197

baby must deal with it by supplying more insulin than normal from its own pancreas. After delivery, when glucose from the mother is no longer present, the baby's pancreas continues to produce insulin. Unless prevented by careful monitoring, the result is hypoglycaemia, which can cause brain damage. A blood glucose level below 3mmol per litre is considered to be hypoglycaemia in the infant.

Confinement The actual delivery of the baby is a time to be carefully evaluated. It is desirable to allow the pregnancy to go near term, if possible, for the health of the baby and particularly for the development of its lungs, but the decision whether or not to deliver the baby before the full period of gestation will depend on the health of the mother, the baby, or both. When the decision is made by the doctor for the time of delivery, the type of delivery will also be decided. The earlier the delivery, the safer it will be for the baby to be delivered by caesarean section. Should the foetus be near the full term, the doctor may induce labour by the infusion of oxytocin, a pituitary hormone. Controversy surrounds the risk of caesarean section versus normal vaginal delivery; however, recent evidence suggests that a normal delivery squeezes the baby's lungs, helping to clear fluid from the airways.

Lactation, or the production of milk in the diabetic mother, means the mother will have to remain on insulin even if she was not insulin-dependent before pregnancy, since oral hypoglycaemic agents pass through to the mother's milk. During lactation, lactose, or milk sugar, may be evident in the urine; it will test positive in a Clinitest but is not picked up by Clinistix; therefore Clinistix should be used for urine testing at this time. Any mother should be encouraged to nurse her baby when possible, as human milk is the food meant for babies, and carries with it protection against disease for the child.

PREMARIN See HORMONES.

PREMATURE Refers to a baby born before it is fully developed (9 months), or one that weighs less than 5 pounds or less than 2,250 grams. See also PREGNANCY AND CHILDBIRTH.

PRENATAL CARE. The care of mother and child before birth.

See also PREGNANCY AND CHILDBIRTH.

PREPUCE   See GENITALIA.

PRESCRIPTION   An order for drugs, diet, or other special treatments from licensed or authorised persons.

PRESSURE SORES   See BED SORES.

PRICKLING   See DIABETIC NEUROPATHY; PARAES-THESIA.

PRIMARY DIABETES   See DIABETES MELLITUS.

PROGNOSIS   A prediction or estimate of what may happen in the course of an illness or a disease.

PROGRESSIVE DISEASE   A disease that cannot be cured, and which worsens in time.

PROINSULIN   See INSULIN.

PROLIFERATION   An increasing or spreading, as in proliferative retinopathy. See RETINA, RETINOPATHY.

PROMPT INSULIN ZINC SUSPENSION   Semilente insulin. See INSULIN.

PROSTHESIS   An artificial part replacing a missing part, such as an artificial leg or eye.

PROSTAGLANDINS   A variety of fatty acid substances that have been found in virtually every tissue and organ system in man. Their various functions include increased exchange of fluids between the blood and other tissues; smooth muscle contraction; bronchial constriction; and alteration of pain thresholds, a mechanism that is not well understood. The greater part of their action appears to be that of a messenger in directing the activities of the cells. See also RESEARCH.

PROTAMINE ZINC INSULIN (PZI)   See INSULIN

PROTEIN   Nitrogen compounds composed of amino acids: a necessary source of food. Protein is equally good whether obtained from an animal or a vegetable source. Vegetable protein, however, must be eaten from a wide variety of foods to include all the essential amino acids. A complete vegetarian diet, one that does not include milk, eggs, or cheese, must be supplemented with vitamin B_{12}. If you are a vegetarian, inform your doctor. Vegetarian Food Exchange lists are included under FOOD EXCHANGES.

All protein yields 4 calories/gram, and is broken down in the digestive process to amino acids for use by the body

199

cells. Protein requirements in the diabetic diet are in dispute, but the general trend is to decrease the percentage of calories from protein and fat and increase carbohydrate (starch). See also ALBUMIN; AMINO ACIDS; CARBOHYDRATE; DIET; FAT; KIDNEY DISEASE; NITROGEN BALANCE.

PROTEIN SYNTHESIS The making of protein by the body for growth and repair of tissue. See also AMINO ACIDS; METABOLISM.

PROTEINURIA Protein in the urine. See also ALBUMIN; KIDNEY DISEASE; URINE TESTS.

PROTOCOL The outline or plan for an experiment, test, or treatment.

PROXIMAL Nearest to the point of attachment. A cut on a toe near where the toe attaches to the foot is proximal to the foot; a cut on the end of the toe near the nail is distal to the foot.

PRURITUS See ITCHING.

PSYCHIATRIST A medical doctor who has had specialised training in the diagnosis, prevention, and treatment of mental and emotional disorders.

PSYCHOLOGIST A specialist trained through extra courses of study to observe, test, and treat behaviour problems. A psychologist has a master's or PhD (doctor of philosophy) degree in psychology, and practices alone or acts as a consultant to a psychiatrist. A psychologist may not, by law, prescribe medication.

PTOSIS Drooping of the eyelid. It is caused by a nervous system disease of the third cranial nerve. See DIABETIC NEUROPATHY; NERVOUS SYSTEM.

PUBERTY See ADOLESCENCE.

PUBLICATIONS FOR DIABETICS See APPENDIX B: COOKBOOKS; APPENDIX C: SUGGESTED READING;

PUERTO RICAN DIET See FOOD EXCHANGES, Exchange Lists for Ethnic Foods.

PULSE As the heart pumps blood through the body, the arteries pulsate with each beat. This can be felt with the fingers, and is most commonly counted over the radial artery on the wrist just beyond the base of the thumb. Feel for the pulse with the fingers, being careful not to press so hard as to shut off the flow of blood. To take a quick count, hold for 15 seconds and multiply by 4. For greater accuracy, count for a full minute, noting if the beat is even or irregular, strong or weak. In a medical emergency, the doctor may ask for this information.

PUS   See INFECTION AND INFLAMMATION.
PYELOGRAM   See INTRAVENOUS PYELOGRAM.
PYELONEPHRITIS   See KIDNEY DISEASE.
PYORRHOEA   See MOUTH CARE.

Q

QUALITATIVE ANALYSIS A test that is concerned with the kind of substance present rather than the amount; for example, to determine what kinds of ketones are present in the urine or blood. See also KETONE BODIES.

QUANTITIVE ANALYSIS A test that is concerned with the amount of a certain substance present rather than the kind. From qualitative analysis above, and using ketones as an example, the test would not be concerned with identifying the types of ketones present, but only the amount.

QUANTITATIVE FAECES COLLECTION See FAT DETERMINATION STOOL COLLECTION.

QUART See METRIC SYSTEM.

QUICK-ACTING CARBOHYDRATES See SUGAR.

R

RADIOIMMUNOASSAY   See IMMUNOASSAY.

RADIOPAQUE DYE   A dye injected into a vein or artery so that blood vessels or organs can be seen on a special X-ray machine. See ANGIOGRAPHY.

RAFFINOSE   See SUGAR.

RANDOM BLOOD SUGAR (RBS), or GLUCOSE (RBG)   See BLOOD TESTS.

RASH   A general term for skin change – usually an eruption of reddish and itchy spots on skin. See ITCHING.

RASTINON   See ORAL HYPOGLYCAEMIC AGENTS.

REACTIVE HYPOGLYCAEMIA   See HYPOGLYCAEMIA.

REAGENT   Any substance involved in a chemical reaction. Examples of reagents are reagent strips and tablets used in urine tests (see).

RECEPTOR SITES   See CELLS; RESEARCH.

RECESSIVE GENE   See CELLS.

RECIPES FOR DIABETICS   APPENDIX B: COOKBOOKS.

RECOMBINANT DNA   See CELLS; RESEARCH.

RECORDS   Keep records of all urine tests and medication taken. Additional records of what you eat and the amount of exercise you take may be helpful. Make note of any hypoglycaemic reactions and when they happen. Your doctor may have a sheet prepared for this, or you can buy a small booklet called a Clinilog produced by the Ames Company. Most pharmacies stock them, or will order them for you.

RECTAL THERMOMETER   See THERMOMETER, CLINICAL.

RECTUM   The lowest part of the digestive tract.

RED BLOOD CELLS (RBC)   See BLOOD.

REDUCING DIET   See DIET.

REFINED SUGAR   Ordinary table sugar. See SUGAR.

REFLECTANCE METER   See EYETONE REFLECTANCE COLORIMETER; RESEARCH.

REFLEX   An action that occurs involuntarily on stimulation.

REGIMEN   A plan to follow as a diet or medical treatment, or both, designed especially to help with a health problem.

REGISTRAR   A physician who continues medical training in order to prepare for certification as a specialist in a given field or area.

REGULAR INSULIN   See SOLUBLE INSULIN.

REMISSION PERIOD   Also known as the honeymoon period, it often occurs in the juvenile-onset type of diabetes mellitus. After initial treatment, and depending on the degree of damage to pancreatic beta cells, the pancreas may begin to produce insulin again. Insulin requirements decrease to very low levels, for weeks, months, or even years. Some doctors discontinue treatment with insulin at this time; however, many feel that simply by decreasing insulin, emotional adjustment to diabetes is more easily effected. Also, the supplementation of the body's own insulin with low-dose injections may prolong the remission period. This is another area of controversy.

RENAL ANGIOGRAPHY   See ANGIOGRAPHY; KIDNEY DISEASE.

RENAL BIOPSY   See KIDNEY DISEASE.

RENAL DISEASE   See KIDNEY DISEASE.

RENAL THRESHOLD   The renal threshold can be compared to a dam holding back substances such as water and glucose to meet the needs of the body. When the blood can carry no more sugar, the kidneys remove the excess, 'spilling' it into the urine. That point varies from person to person, but 10 mmol per litre is the norm. Pregnant diabetics and those with juvenile-onset diabetes can have a renal threshold as low as 6.7 mmol per litre, while older diabetics are known to have a threshold of 12 mmol per litre or higher. See also DIABETES MELLITUS, JUVENILE-ONSET; KIDNEYS; PREGNANCY AND CHILDBIRTH; RESEARCH; URINE TESTS.

RENAL TRANSPLANTS   See RESEARCH.

REPLACEMENT THERAPY   Substitute treatment for something that is lacking. When a person has little or no insulin available to supply the needs of the body, insulin or beta cell stimulants (ORAL HYPOGLYCAEMIC AGENTS) are given as replacement therapy.

RESEARCH   To this date diabetes remains a disease not only without a cure, but also in some cases with questions as to its cause (see DIABETES MELLITUS). Only recently have funds been made available in amounts that will make possible some of the much-needed research.

Insulin can correct the life-threatening emergency of diabetic ketoacidosis as well as permitting patients with diabetes to lead productive lives. It cannot, however, cure the disease or prevent the ultimate development of the long-term complications of this affliction.

Scientists in many disciplines are involved in diabetes research that is yielding new information about the causes of diabetes, new methods of treatment, and new techniques for the study of the basic mechanisms resulting in the complications of diabetes. Of the hundreds of research projects currently funded, only general areas of research will be discussed.

For convenience, the areas are divided into five sections. General highlights of research activity are given without specific details of the research procedures.

Causes of Diabetes   Recent collaborative studies involving specialists in diabetes, genetics, immunology and virology have gathered data suggesting that viral infections, possibly with common viruses like the mumps and measles viruses, may result in extensive damage of pancreatic cells and thereby cause diabetes. This may be particularly true of juvenile-onset diabetes, in which children with certain genetic backgrounds may be more susceptible to virus infection, which may then lead to extensive damage to the pancreas. More than twenty-six different viruses have been implicated. Genetic patterns are seen with greater frequency in juvenile diabetes than in the general population.

Using certain strains of mice, researchers have now shown that several types of viruses that affect the brain and heart cells can also infect and destroy the pancreatic islets. Other strains of mice are resistant to the same virus infection. When cells from mice are grown in culture, it has been observed that the genetic makeup of the different strains of cells determines whether the virus can or cannot attach to the cell surface, with subsequent penetration and damage to the cell.

If, indeed, specific viral agents can be shown to be the cause of juvenile-onset diabetes, then preventive viral vacines could be produced that would give juveniles active immunity.

Recent studies indicate that the genetic factors associated with the development of adult-onset diabetes are different from the genetic factors seen in juvenile-onset diabetes.

Cures for Diabetes   Insulin has permitted patients with diabetes to lead productive lives, but it has not cured diabetes. For many diabetics, the treatment regimens with insulin may delay, but not prevent, the eventual development of the complications of diabetes that account for the high mortality and morbidity rates associated with the disease.

Using highly inbred strains of mice, researchers have shown that it is possible to transplant pancreatic islets to cure diabetes. The exciting prospect of transplanting pancreas cells in humans is complicated by, first, the difficulty of growing these cells in culture, and second, the destruction of the transplanted tissue by the immune system of the individual who has received the transplant. Transplant rejection can be decreased by the use of drugs that suppress the immune mechanism, but for the diabetic this brings about further complications of infection and metabolic changes.

The combined efforts of immunologists, cell biologists, and biochemists working in the areas of tissue culture and transplantation immunology may in the future make it possible to transplant isolated pancreatic islets as a means of curing diabetes.

For those diabetics with failing kidneys, kidney transplants continue. Thousands of kidney transplants are on record. Sources of kidneys for transplant are made available through signed permission from the persons who wish to donate their organs after death, and from living volunteers. One healthy kidney is adequate to sustain normal human life. Every attempt is made to obtain a kidney from persons whose tissues match as closely as possible, because tissue rejection continues to plague kidney transplantation, and the programme must continue as a research project.

Complications of Diabetes Researchers have been investigating the mechanisms of diabetes complications for years. The long-term complications of diabetes mellitus are usually grouped into two categories: (1) large-vessel disease, or macroangiopathy – a disorder related to the fast rate of fatty deposits in the large arteries – and (2) small-vessel disease, or microangiopathy – a disorder associated with changes in the small blood vessels in the body, the capillaries. The diabetic is more susceptible to those two disorders than is the nondiabetic.

1. The development of atherosclerosis – fatty deposits on the arterial walls – is much higher in persons with diabetes; it accounts for the three- to fourfold increased risk of heart attacks that diabetics suffer when compared at any age with the nondiabetic population. Investigators have been able to examine the tissue layers of the arterial wall and have noted in detail the changes that take place with varying diets, hormonal factors, and blood components. Recent studies have shown that certan lipoproteins interact with different cellular materials of the vessel wall and may start a sequence of events that could finally lead to and speed up the atherosclerotic process. Research has also shown that there are changes in the metabolism of arterial wall tissues of diabetic experimental animals; a high blood glucose level bathing these tissues is particularly involved in these changes.

Research is being carried out on the alterations in the function of the platelets in diabetics. Platelets are one of the cellular portions of blood specifically involved in the clotting mechanism. These investigations include the prostaglandins, which are synthesised in platelets, and also the cells lining the inner surface of blood vessels (endothelial cells); the prostaglandins have been shown to be important control hormones of the coagulation process.

2. Small blood vessel complications of diabetes have been associated with the thickening of capillary basement membrane, which probably interferes with the movement of nutrients to the tissues and the removal of the waste products of cell metabolism. New techniques have been developed to isolate the capillary membrane and analyse its

chemical structure. Evidence indicates that the membrane in diabetic patients has a chemically different composition from that seen in normal individuals.

Further research suggests that other metabolic defects unique to the tissues of diabetics may play an important role in the lesions that occur as complications of the disease. Findings also indicate that exposure of the arterial wall, peripheral nerves, or the lens of the eye to high blood glucose levels results in the collection of certain compounds; these in turn distrupt the biochemistry of these tissues, leading to functional and structural disturbances. A real breakthrough came when techniques were developed enabling scientists to grow, in the laboratory, lens tissue, retinal capillaries, cellular components of the kidney, and various nerve cells. This allows for the development of model systems to distinguish between genetically controlled (primary) factors and poor control of blood glucose levels (secondary factors) that may lead to diabetic complications; further understanding of the distinctions will permit the development of treatments to correct specific defects.

Research in another area has occupied the attention of investigators in the past decade. It is the recognition that the cell (plasma) membrane surrounding cells is a complex structure that controls the passage of nutrients into the cell and waste products out of the cell and that is also possesses the specific receptors that interact with numerous substances such as antigens, antibodies, and hormones. Currently techniques are being used to purify cell membrane insulin receptors to study their chemistry, structure, and function.

Treatment and Control of Diabetes There is no doubt that one of the most controversial aspects of diabetes research has been that associated with genetic engineering or molecular engineering – the research dealing with recombinant DNA. Clones and cloning are words seen frequently in newspapers and magazines over the last few years. A clone is a family of cells that are the product of a single cell that has multiplied by binary fission. (*Binary fission* is the splitting of one cell into two equal parts each containing the same genetic material as the original cell.) All the cells in a clone are therefore genetically identical. Researchers are attempting to turn certain bacteria (*Escherichia coli,* or *E. coli* for short) into microscopic drug factories by altering their genetic structure with a process of splitting their DNA loops and recombining the DNA with certain added genes (see CELLS). This is called recombinant DNA. The hope is that *E. coli* or some other bacterium can be genetically altered to produce insulin identical to human insulin.

Progress has been made in developing and testing devices that can monitor the blood glucose and then administer insulin. The Biostator Glucose Controlled Insulin Infusion System (Life Science Instruments, Miles Laboratories, Inc.) is a bedside machine about the size of a large portable television set that has been developed as a research tool. Although not everyone is convinced that the maintenance of blood glucose at normal or near levels can prevent, reduce, or even reverse the complications of diabetes, it has been shown that pregnant diabetics who were monitored by the machine had fewer complications of pregnancy and bore healthier babies.

A number of investigators have demonstrated the effectiveness of photocoagulation in slowing the progression of vision-threatening retinopathy. See RETINA, RETINOPATHY.

The home monitoring of glucose with the use of the Enzyme Reflectance Colorimeter (Ames Company) with Dextrostix and a similar meter Glucocheck (Medistron) has been effective and practical, with and without the reflectance meters, in helping the diabetic to gain better control.

Haemoglobin A_1 A family of haemoglobin molecules (the red pigment in blood) which have become chemically combined with glucose (glycosylated). The best known is called haemoglobin A_{1C}. The level of this in the blood, expressed as a percentage of the total haemoglobin, depends upon the average level of blood glucose in the preceding few weeks. The higher the percentage, the worse the control. In non-diabetics, the level of haemoglobin A_{1C} is between 2% and 7%. In well controlled diabetics it is between 7% and 9%, but when long-term control has been bad it may be as high as 20%. Measurement of haemoglobin A_1 or A_{1C} is being used increasingly to gauge long-term control and seems to be more useful than the occasional estimation of blood glucose concentration.

Somatostatin, a potent hormone produced by the hypothalamus and various other tissues, including the delta cells of the pancreas, has now been synthesised in the laboratory. Somatostatin was first named because it suppresses growth hormone (somatotropin or somatotrophin). It also suppresses glucagon and insulin. Exactly how somatostatin works is not clear; it appears to suppress glucagon more than it suppresses insulin, and thus it has been useful in diabetes when high blood glucose and high blood ketones are caused by an excess of glucagon and a deficiency of insulin. Long-term administration of somatostatin needs further research.

Finally, some progress is being made in an attempt to deliver insulin by the oral route. Tiny packages made of fat, called liposomes, may make it possible to carry insulin safely past the digestive juices of the stomach, thus eliminating the need for injections. There are many difficulties to overcome, among them, the absorption of liposomal insulin from the gut.

Behavioural and Psychosocial Research in Diabetes At present there is no large-scale research being conducted in this important area of diabetes. Physicians, nurses, parents, and all diabetes-supporting personnel are concerned about the frequency with which psychosocial difficulties interfere with the therapy and daily-life patterns of the diabetic, particularly of the young insulin-dependent diabetic.

Funding for this kind of research has been lacking as has also the interest by investigators.

RESPIRATION Respiration is more than breathing in and out; it is involved with the release of oxygen and the removal of carbon dioxide at the cell level, called cellular or tissue respiration. See also CELLS; METABOLISM.

RESPIRATORY ACIDOSIS An acid-base imbalance; a fall in arterial blood or plasma pH to less than 7.35, and a rise in plasma carbon dioxide (CO_2) to greater than 30 millimoles per litre. Whenever breathing is impaired by injury, disease, or poisoning, the lungs cannot rid the body of carbon dioxide. The excess CO_2 is picked up by the blood; it combines with hydrogen and water to form carbonic acid ($H_2O + CO_2 \rightarrow H_2CO_3$), which lowers the blood pH. Symptoms of respiratory acidosis start with drowsiness, and proceed to stupor and coma. See also ACID-BASE BALANCE; COMA.

RESPIRATORY ALKALOSIS An acid-base imbalance; a rise in arterial blood or plasma pH to greater than 7.45 and a fall in plasma carbon dioxide (CO_2) to less than 24 millimoles per litre. Respiratory alkalosis is usually caused by breathing too fast, but it can also be caused by poisons, especially those in the aspirin family (salicylates). Symptoms include numbness and tingling (paraesthesia), lightheadedness, agitation, and fainting. See also ACID-BASE BALANCE.

RESPIRATORY DISTRESS SYNDROME (RDS) Breathing difficulties in infants. Se also PREGNANCY AND CHILDBIRTH.

RESTAURANTS See DIET; FOOD EXCHANGES FOR FAST FOOD RESTAURANTS.

RETICULOENDOTHELIAL SYSTEM See LYMPH, LYMPHATIC SYSTEM.

RETINA, RETINOPATHY The retina is the light-sensitive centre at the back of the eye. When the doctor examines your eye with a light (ophthalmoscope), he is looking at the retina for signs of disease, called retinopathy. The retina is served by many tiny blood vessels and is covered with nerve cells connecting the optic nerve to the brain. Damage to these cells impairs vision. Not all diabetics have retinopathy, but many do, and the progression of this disease is related to high blood glucose. There is evidence that control of blood glucose in the early stages of diabetes may prevent or slow down retinopathy, but once retinopathy is established, control of the blood glucose may not help appreciably. There are several main events in diabetic retinopathy as follows:

Macular Oedema The macula lutea is a point of clearest vision on the retina. Fluid, or oedema, in this area dims the vision.

Vitreous Haemorrhage The blood vessels of the retina may enlarge into tiny balloonlike sacs called microaneurysms, which may break open, and haemorrhage, causing damage to the retina. A spreading of haemorrhages on the retina and into the vitreous fluid of the eyeball is called vitreous haemorrhage. The vitreous fluid occupies most of the area of the eyeball and gives it a round shape. When leaking blood clouds the vitreous fluid, an operation called a vitrectomy can be performed. A surgeon makes a tiny slit in the eyeball and removes the clouded fluid, replacing it with a salt solution.

Retinal Detachment When haemorrhages occur, the body responds by providing new blood vessels. This is called neovascularisation. These new blood vessels tend to be pulled away from the retina by the force of vitreous shrinking, causing further haemorrhage and retinal detachment.

Exudates Sometimes found on the retina of the eye; their presence may be the first sign that the patient has diabetes. There are two kinds: cotton-wool or soft exudates, which are thought to be formed in areas where the blood supply has been cut off; and waxy or hard exudates, which are high in protein and fat. Lipaemia retinalis, or fat deposits on the retina, is caused by high triglyceride levels; it disappears with the return to normal blood triglycerides. See also LIPIDS.

Glaucoma A disease of the eye somewhat more prevalent in the diabetic than in the nondiabetic population; it involves increased pressure within the eyeball. Always report blurred vision, or coloured circles, especially around lights, to the doctor. Early detection can be treated with drugs. Glaucoma that occurs as a result of neovascularisation, for reasons that are not understood, usually has a sudden onset featuring severe eye pain. This type of glaucoma does not respond well to either medical or surgical treatment.

Tests Tests for the presence of eye disease include electroretinography to check nerve response on the retina, and ultrasonography, which uses harmless sound waves to chart areas of damage in the eye. (See ULTRASONOGRAPHY.) Also, the pupils of the eye can be dilated by medicated drops, a harmless and painless procedure. When the pupils are dilated, the doctor has a much larger window through which to view the retina, and with the use of a very powerful light, he can make an estimate for any damage, and decide what other tests may be necessary, or what treatment is best.

Treatment   Microaneurysms and haemorrhages can be treated with photocoagulation, in which laser beams change light into heat; the heat destroys the small ballooning blood vessels to prevent their rupture or seals off vessels that are already bleeding. Waxy exudates are treated by change to a low-fat diet featuring polyunsaturated fats and weight loss if indicated. See also LIPIDS; RESEARCH.

Pituitary Ablation   The removal of the front or anterior lobe of the pituitary gland. Some doctors feel this procedure slows down the spread of retinal disease and improves vision. This is used as a last resort when all other treatments have failed. See also BLINDNESS; EYESIGHT. *Smoking is thought to worsen blood vessel disease of the retina.*

RETROGRADE EJACULATION   The passage of seminal fluid into the urinary bladder instead of being ejaculated from the penis. See DIABETIC NEUROPATHY.

RETROGRADE RADIOGRAPHY   See KIDNEY DISEASE.

REUSABLE, or GLASS, SYRINGES   See INSULIN SYRINGES AND THEIR CARE.

RIBONUCLEIC ACID (RNA)   See CELLS.

RNIB   Royal National Institute for the Blind. (See Directory.) This body can advise on low vision aids, Braille and talking books.

ROTATION of INJECTION SITES   See INSULIN INJECTION AND INJECTION SITES.

ROUGHAGE   See FIBRE.

RUBBING ALCOHOL   See ALCOHOL; ALCOHOL SWABS.

RUBELLA   See MEASLES.

RUM   See ALCOHOL.

S

SACCHARIDES   One of a series of carbohydrates, including the sugars. The saccharides are divided into monosaccharides, disaccharides, trisaccharides, and polysaccharides, according to the number of saccharide groups comprising them. See CARBOHYDRATES; SUGARS.

SACCHARIN   See Sugar Substitutes under SUGAR.

SALICYLATES   A group of commonly used pain-killing and fever-reducing (antipyretic) drugs: aspirin (acetyl salicylic acid), also called ASA; sodium salicylate; methyl salicylate (oil of wintergreen); and salicylic acid.

Aspirin is used extensively as a pain killer and antipyretic. It is not as safe a drug as commonly thought, because it can cause bleeding and tinnitus (ringing in the ears), is irritating to the stomach, and causes salicylate poisoning in high dosages, especially among children. Aspirin is used in combination with many other drugs. Be sure to read labels. Diabetics taking oral hypoglycaemic agents should be aware that aspirin may decrease the blood glucose, thus increasing the effect of these drugs. Large doses of aspirin can cause falsely high readings on urine tests when using Clinitest tablets, Clinistix, and Diastix.

Sodium salicylate is used less often than aspirin and, while not as strong, has the same general effect.

Oil of wintergreen is used topically (on the skin) only. It can cause poisoning in children if applied too liberally and too often.

Mild salicylate poisoning, called salicylism, presents symptoms that include nausea and vomiting, ringing in the ears (very common), dizziness, problems with vision and hearing, sweating, and diarrhoea. Serious salicylate poisoning includes coma, irregular pulse, changes in blood pressure (first a rise, then a fall), and increased respirations (see RESPIRATORY ALKALOSIS). Some people are very sensitive to salicylates. Death can result in those with an allergy

214

(hypersensitivity) to aspirin. See ALLERGY.

Substitutes for aspirin should be discussed with your doctor. Many doctors recommend the use of paracetamol which can be bought under that generic name, or under the trade name of Panadol. Some pain-killer compounds feature a mixture of aspirin and paracetamol.

SALT   See SODIUM.

SALT SUBSTITUES   See SODIUM.

SATIETY   Condition of sufficiency, being satisfied after a meal and not needing or wanting more food. Satiety is not well understood.

SATURATED FATS AND OILS   See LIPIDS.

SAUCES   Stay away from sauces unless you know what is in them. They can be made at home using food exchanges from your diet plan.

SCALES   See DIET SCALE.

SCLEROSIS   A hardening or thickening of tissue. See also HEART DISEASE.

SEASONINGS   See CONDIMENTS; FOOD FLAVOURING; Salt Substitutes under SODIUM; Sugar Substitutes under SUGAR.

SEASICKNESS   Motion sickness. See TRAVELLING WITH DIABETES.

SECONDARY DIABETES   See DIABETES MELLITUS.

SECONDARY HYPERTENSION   See BLOOD PRESSURE.

SECOND-VOIDED URINE SPECIMENS   See URINE TESTS.

SECRETE   To produce a substance and to release it; for example, digestive juices are secreted from the pancreas into the small intestine. See also GLANDS.

SEDENTARY   Sitting down; not moving about. See also INACTIVITY; SKIN CARE.

SEIZURES   A sudden onset of pain or a series of uncontrollable muscle spasms (a convulsion). A seizure can happen to anyone suffering from injury, heatstroke, poisoning, disease, alcoholism, or a high fever. Although rare, low blood glucose can also cause a seizure.

In case of a seizure, turn the victim on his side to prevent vomitus from getting into his lungs. In hospitals where a seizure is anticipated, padded tongue blades are taped to the bed for use to place between the teeth to protect the tongue. At home, however, there is usually no time to do this, and if something other than this is used, the victim may break his teeth or bite the substitute into pieces, further complicating the situation. Do not try to give him fluids or food until he is fully awake. See also HYPOGLYCAEMIC REACTIONS; GLUCAGON.

SEMILENTE INSULIN See INSULIN.

SEMINAL FLUID Fluid carrying semen through the urethra of the penis during ejaculation. See also RETROGRADE EJACULATION.

SENSITIVITY See ALLERGY.

SENSORY LOSS See DIABETIC NEUROPATHY: PARAES-THESIA: SKIN CARE.

SERUM See BLOOD.

SERUM ALBUMIN See ALBUMIN; BLOOD TESTS.

SERUM CHOLESTEROL See BLOOD TESTS; LIPIDS.

SERUM GLUCOSE See GLUCOSE.

SEVENTY-TWO-HOUR FAST In the fasting state, glucose is produced by the liver from protein and fat in a process called gluconeogenesis, and the supply of insulin should decrease. If it does not decrease, the fast then indicates oversecretion or hypersecretion of insulin, perhaps caused by a tumour. Moderate exercise may be ordered during the three-day fast. Blood will be drawn at intervals. If there is a hypoglycaemic reaction, blood will also be drawn for testing. See also TUMOURS.

SEX HORMONES See HORMONES.

SEX ORGANS See GENITALIA.

SEXUAL INTERCOURSE Usually the desire for sexual intercourse is unchanged in both the male and female diabetic, but blood vessel disease or nervous system disease (diabetic neuropathy) may make it impossible for the male to gain an erection. It has also been reported that about 30 per cent of diabetic women under the age of 45, when compared to nondiabetics, suffered a loss of orgasmic response. It is not known to what degree the loss of sexual function can be attributed to psychological or to other stress factors. See also IMPOTENCE.

SHAKING Tremors, or shaking of part or parts of the body, may be a sign of low blood glucose. See also HYPOGLY-CAEMIC REACTIONS.

SHEETBURN   See BED SORES.

SHELLFISH   See FOOD EXCHANGES, List 5 (Lean Meat).

SHIN SPOTS   See SKIN DISEASES.

SHOCK   A state of collapse. In diabetics, shock is sometimes used in the same sense as coma, as in insulin shock. See also ALLERGY; HYPOGLYCAEMIC REACTIONS.

SHOES   See FEET, CARE OF.

SHORT-ACTING INSULIN   Soluble insulin. See INSULIN.

SHOTS   See INSULIN INJECTION AND INJECTION SITES.

SICKNESS   Everyone gets sick once in a while, but when a diabetic gets sick, diabetes is harder to control because sickness is a stress to the body. In addition, sickness may be accompanied by a decrease in both activity and appetite. Inactivity changes the rate at which the body utilises food and usually increases the need for insulin. A decrease in appetite will have various effects. Nausea, vomiting, and diarrhoea may further inhibit the intake of food; nevertheless, it is important for the patient to eat and to continue to take insulin or other diabetic medication. Ideally, the doctor should discuss the steps to be taken in the event of sickness, but too often this is not done, and the patient is left to his own judgement or that of his family.

First, if you are sick, check your urine before each meal and at bedtime for sugar and acetone. Take your temperature and keep a record of all tests, elevation of temperature, and the amount of food, and insulin, or pills, taken. Follow the plan set up by your doctor in case of sickness; however, if you are unable to control your blood glucose, contact him with the information you have recorded. Diabetes can worsen within a matter of hours. If you cannot get in touch with your doctor, gather your records and get someone to take you to the nearest hospital. (If no one is available, call a taxi.)

Diabetics who take insulin may need to change the dosage; those who take oral hypoglycaemic agents or who are controlled by diet alone may need insulin temporarily during illness or other stress. If your doctor prescribes insulin, see INSULIN, INSULIN SYRINGES AND THEIR care; INSULIN INJECTION AND INJECTION SITES. Those who are already using insulin and need to increase the dosage may follow a general rule suggested by Luther B. Travis, MD, in *An Instructional Aid on Juvenile Diabetes Mellitus.** Dr Travis recommends increasing the amount of insulin by about 10 per cent; for example, if you are taking 30 units of NPH insulin, increase it to 33 units. Again, a note of caution: Talk this over with your doctor in advance, and never decrease or increase an insulin dosage drastically without a doctor's order. It is also a good idea to have soluble insulin on hand at all times in case the doctor wants you to use it as a supplement.

Should you become sick and your urine tests show no sugar, *do not* increase your insulin; your blood glucose may be too low. If you have Dextrostix (see BLOOD TESTS), test your blood glucose or call the doctor for a laboratory appointment for testing. Any symptoms of a hypoglycaemic reaction should be treated with sugar in some form. (See HYPOGLYCAEMIC REACTIONS.) Persistent symptoms of this nature indicate that you probably need to decrease the amount of insulin. Again, the decrease is usually about 10 per cent**; for example, 30 units of insulin should be decreased to 27 units. The diabetic must assume responsibility for his own care to a great extent; however, things must never get out of hand. The doctor is there to help when you need it; *when in doubt, consult him.*

For treatment of motion sickness, see TRAVELLING WITH DIABETES.

Sick-day diet rules as follows are adapted from the Kaiser Permanente Diet Manual.*** Go over these meal plans with your doctor for his approval.

Diet During Sickness   If, because of sickness, you are unable to follow your daily meal plan, you should replace at least the carbohydrate allowance for each meal. This may be done by using liquid food such as juices, milk, soups, or hot cereals, depending on what you can tolerate.

*See Appendix D: Emergencies
**Recommended by Dr Travis (see above)
***Used with the permission of Mary E. Wilson, RD, former Clinical Dietitian, Kaiser Permanente Medical Group Clinic, Fontana, California.

Diabetics who are insulin dependent should have a minimum of 150 grams of carbohydrate each day while sick.

The following suggested meal plans may be used during an acute sickness; they contain between 150 and 160 grams of carbohydrate. Suggested times are given for taking fluids; however, you may alter the times to meet your own needs. One cup is 8 ounces, or 240 millitres.

MEAL PLAN I

160 grams carbohydrate totalling 640 calories

1 cup unsweetened apple or orange juice, regular ginger ale, or 7-Up as first nourishment on arising and every two hours, for a total of eight times a day. For example, if the first juice is taken at 8.00 A.M., the last juice would be taken at 10.00 P.M.

MEAL PLAN II

40 grams protein, 5 grams fat, 150 grams
carbohydrate totaling 805 calories

Some nourishment is to be taken every two hours starting at 8.00 A.M., or whatever hour the patient awakens in the morning.

8.00 A.M.	1 cup unsweetened orange or apple juice.
	Eggnog made with: 1 cup skim milk; 1 egg
	(soft-coddle before whipping into milk); 1 teaspoon
	sugar; and vanilla to taste
10.00 A.M.	½ cup beef broth
12.00 NOON	1 cup skim milk
2.00 P.M.	1 cup regular ginger ale or 7-Up
4.00 P.M.	1 cup unsweetened orange or apple juice
6.00 P.M.	½ cup chicken broth
	1 cup skim milk
8.00 P.M.	¾ cup grape juice
10.00 P.M.	Cocoa (unsweetened type) made with:
	1 cup skim milk and 1 teaspoon sugar

MEAL PLAN III

55 grams protein, 20 grams fat, 155 grams carbohydrate
totalling, 1,020 calories

Some nourishment is to be taken every two hours starting at 8.00 A.M. or whatever hour the patient awakens in the morning.

8.00 A.M.	1 cup unsweetened orange or apple juice.
	½ cup cooked cereal
	½ cup skim milk
10.00 A.M.	Eggnog (see Meal Plan II)
12.00 NOON	1 cup strained cream soup
	½ cup skim milk
	½ cup vanilla ice cream (regular)
2.00 P.M.	½ cup unsweetened orange juice
4.00 P.M.	1 cup skim milk
6.00 P.M.	1 cup strained cream soup
	1 cup skim milk
8.00 P.M.	1 cup unsweetened orange juice
10.00 P.M.	1 cup skim milk

SIDE EFFECTS   Any effect from a drug that is not the one for which the drug was ordered. Examples of common side effects are skin rashes, nausea, vomiting, diarrhoea, and alterations in test results. Some side effects are predictable, and the doctor will caution against them. For instance, the antibiotic Keflin (IV or IM) or Keflex (oral) can produce discoloration of urine tests done with Clinitest tablets. If, however, you feel you are experiencing an unwanted or disturbing side effect, let the doctor know immediately because this may mean that you are hypersensitive to that drug. This is known also as an untoward reaction, such as difficulty in breathing, welts in the skin, or itching of the skin, inside the mouth or throat, or a change in the action of the heart. See also ALLERGY; INHIBITOR; POTENTIATION.

SIGHT   See EYESIGHT.

SIMPLE LIPIDS   See LIPIDS.

SIMPLE SUGARS   See SUGAR.

SINGLE COMPONENT INSULIN AND SINGLE PEAK INSULIN   See INSULIN.

SITE   See INSULIN INJECTION AND INJECTION SITES.

SKIM MILK   See FOOD EXCHANGES, List 1.

SKIN CARE   The skin is a covering organ containing pores, which aid in the elimination of waste materials; nerves, which notify the person of environmental danger; and sweat glands, which aid in the regulation of body temperature. Sweating for no apparent reason may be a sign of low blood glucose. If the skin is hot, take your temperature; it may be a warning that you are sick. (See THERMOMETER, CLINICAL.) Most people do not take proper care of the skin, unless their skin is extra sensitive to the sun or to certain foods or drugs. The skin reflects the care it is given and the person's general state of health. See also BED SORES; BURNS; FEET, CARE OF; HANDS.

SKIN DISEASES   The skin is the first line of defence against infection. Athlete's foot, *Candida albicans,* and gangrene are all more prevalent when diabetes is in poor control.

Shin Spots are brown spots occurring on the shins related to blood vessel disease. They occur more frequently in males, and with increased frequency in diabetes of long duration. At first the lesions are dull, flat, red papules 5 to 12 mm (¼ to ½″) in diameter, becoming brownish. They are not painful, usually give no trouble, and require no treatment.

Necrobiosis Lipoidica Diabeticorum appears as single or multiple lesions on the thighs, arms, hands, abdomen, breast, back, and most often on the shins and ankles – in females more often than in males. Fortunately, this is a rare complication. The main problem is secondary infection. The lesions may fade in time.

Vitiligo is a loss of pigmentation which appears as whitish patches on the skin. It occurs more frequently in females, and is more common after the age of 40.

Xanthelasmas are yellowish plaques associated with high cholesterol levels in about half the cases. They seem to occur more frequently in diabetics. The lesions can be surgically removed if they are a cosmetic problem, especially on the eyelids and around the eyes. They do not disappear with the lowering of cholesterol.

Xanthomatosis is associated with high triglyceride levels and with diabetes poorly controlled over a long period of time.

These red-yellow lesions appear on various parts of the body – knees, thighs, buttocks – but most often on the elbows, and tend to disappear slowly with a decrease in triglycerides and good diabetic control. See LIPIDS.

SKIN DOCTOR   See DERMATOLOGIST.

SKIN-FOLD MEASUREMENTS   See WEIGHT.

SLEEPING PILLS   Do not take any sleeping pills unless your doctor has advised it. Do not borrow them from friends or buy nonprescription drugs over the counter. *Heavy sleep caused by sleeping pills may cause a hypoglycaemic reaction to go unnoticed.* The sleeping pill chloral hydrate can change the colour of a Clinitest.

SLIDING-SCALE INSULIN COVERAGE   A method of pre-scribing insulin dosage sometimes used in hospitals:

For example

Urine test results	Insulin dosage
4+ urine (glucose)	15 units soluble insulin
3+ urine	10 units soluble insulin
2+ urine	5 units soluble insulin
1+ urine	no insulin

Give 5 units of soluble insulin in addition to the above if acetone is present.

Using a scale such as this means that the patient often is given too much insulin for several reasons:

1. Incorrect testing procedures.
2. Failure to obtain a second-voided specimen (see URINE TESTS).
3. Errors in medication.
4. Reliance on urine test for glucose, which is not a sensitive enough test on which to base insulin dosage.

When too much insulin is given, the blood glucose drops too low, causing an insulin reaction, then no insulin is given and the blood glucose goes back up. The patient bounces up and down between high and low blood glucose; hence the name rebound phenomenon. It is also called the Somogyi effect after the physiologist who first described it. It is hoped that doctors will abandon the use of the sliding-scale insulin coverage and depend on frequent blood testing to regulate insulin dosage.

SNACKS See DIET; FOOD EXCHANGES.

SOCIAL SECURITY BENEFITS If you are disabled and cannot work, whatever your age, and have been paying social security taxes, you may qualify for benefits. Of course, all persons are eligible at the age of 65 if they have been paying social security taxes. Call the nearest social security office, to determine eligibility.

SODA TOP See SOFT DRINKS.

SODIUM (Na) An element and a prominent electrolyte in the body. The amount of fluid in extracellular tissues – tissues not of the blood stream or cells – is largely dependent on the amount of sodium present, because sodium helps retain fluid in these tissues. Normally, fluid balance is regulated by the pumping activity of the heart and by the kidneys, which regulate the amount of sodium in the body. When these fail, as may happen in the complications of diabetes, fluid is retained in the tissues, a condition called oedema. The medical treatment for oedema is to reduce the amount of sodium in the diet, administer diuretics or water pills and, in severe cases, limit fluid intake.

The commonly called 'low-salt diet' is more correctly termed a low-sodium diet. Table salt, or sodium chloride (NaCl, is approximately 40 per cent sodium. (1 teaspoon contains about 2 grams – 2,000 mg – of sodium.) Nevertheless, you will hear the term low-salt diet from most doctors and nurses, because the reduction in the use of table salt is the most common restriction imposed on the person who must limit his intake of sodium.

The average adult American consumes 2,000 to 7,000 mg of sodium daily. This is equal to 6,000 to 18,000 mg of table salt. Table salt is only one source of sodium in the diet. Certain foods naturally contain sodium, but sodium is also added to processed food. Water varies a great deal in the amount of sodium present, depending on the locale; persons on a sodium-restricted diet should avoid the use of water from a water softener (which has a high sodium content) as a drink or in the preparation of food – including ice cubes and tea or coffee. Soft drinks may be high in sodium either because they are made with water having a high sodium content, or because sodium saccharin is added as an artifical sweetener, or sodium citrate as a flavouring. Sodium is found in many drugs such as Alka-Seltzer, and the old home remedy for upset stomach, plain baking soda (sodium bicarbonate), and therefore they should not be used with a sodium-restricted diet. Baking powder that does not contain sodium is available in the dietetic section of the supermarkets. When in doubt about a drug, ask a pharmacist.

The sodium content of food varies, depending on its source. Meat, seed oils, cereal grains, fruits, and most vegetables do not contain significant amounts of sodium (one exception is celery) unless salt or other sodium compounds are added in their preparation or processing. One food additive in particular, monosodium glutamate (MSG), a flavour enhancer, is widely used in many foods. It is added not only to food for home consumption, but also to restaurant foods, especially those serving Chinese food. Meat tenderiser, high in sodium, is also used in many restaurants as is salt in general. All labels must be carefully read for salt (sodium) content. The label on at least one brand of peanut butter states there is no salt added, but further inspection indicates sodium is listed on the nutritional label.

Low-sodium food is found in the dietetic food section of the supermarket; however, 'low sodium' does not mean the food is low in sugar or other calories. Sodium-free bread, butter and margarine are found in the frozen food section. Prepared 'dietetic' foods tend to be expensive. Some alternatives include home baking with sodium-free ingredients (such as sodium-free baking powder); using fresh vegetables and frozen foods prepared without sodium compounds; and rinsing canned vegetables in plain water to rid them of excess salt used in their preparation.

Sodium restricted diets start with severe restrictions, permitting 250 to 500 mg sodium a day for seriously ill patients with gross oedema related to congestive heart failure. Since such a person will be hospitalised, the diet is prepared along guidelines outlined by a registered dietitian, using salt-free bread and butter, only about 4 ounces of cooked meat, a limit on eggs, and an accent on fruit and vegetables. Salt-free milk is obtainable, but the most severely restricted diet will also have a limit on the total fluids permitted in each 24-hour period including any intravenous fluids as determined by the doctor. A sodium-restricted diet of less than 1,000 mg may include some regular bread. A moderately restricted sodium diet, containing 1,000 to 2,000 mg sodium a day, allows regular bread and butter. A mildly restricted sodium diet, with 2,000 to 3,000 mg sodium a day, excludes all highly salted food and the use of salt at the table, but allows meats and vegetables to be lightly salted during preparation.

Diet lists are given to patients by their doctors or dietitians under a doctor's order.

Salt Substitutes An important part of a low-sodium diet; prepared from potassium and ammonium chlorides. A number of salt substitutes are available in supermarkets and pharmacies. Though it is a matter of personal taste, check with your doctor. The secret in using a salt substitute is to add it to food after cooking and to use it sparingly. Carry your salt substitute in your purse or pocket in a small screw-top container. Warn friends who ask you to dinner to leave salt out of the food. Restaurants can do this for you, especially if requested ahead of time. Lastly, do not forget about other flavourings . . . a little dillweed on a hamburger, a little curry on some fish . . . you may find you don't need any salt at all! See also CONDIMENTS; FOOD FLAVOURINGS.

Some High-Sodium Foods to Avoid
Bacon and ham
Canned salmon and tuna
Canned soups
Celery flakes, seed, salt
Chili sauce
Corned beef and pastrami
Cured luncheon meats including frankfurters and
    sausage
Garlic salt and other seasoned salts
Gravies
Horseradish prepared with salt
Instant vegetable broth and packaged dried soups
Ketchup
Meat extracts and tenderisers

Monosodium glutamate (MSG)
Mustard, prepared
Olives, pickles
Parsley flakes
Peanut butter
Potato chips, corn chips, and pretzels
Relishes
Salt
Salted crackers
Salted nuts
Sardines
Sauerkraut
Soy sauce
Tomato paste and sauce
Worcestershire sauce

Most sugar substitutes come in the form of sodium saccharin, which may need to be avoided if you are on a very low-sodium diet. However, saccharin is also available as calcium saccharin. See also Sugar Substitutes under SUGAR.

SODIUM ASCORBATE   See VITAMIN C.

SOFT DIET   See DIET.

SOFT DRINKS (Tonic, Soda Pop)   All soft drinks, except diet drinks, are loaded with sugar; for example, a small 6-ounce bottle of Coca-Cola contains 73 calories and 18 grams of carbohydrate. 7-Up is about the same. Cola and some other soft drinks also contain caffeine, which raises the blood glucose. Drink only diet soda unless you work out a plan with the doctor to include a nondiet type of cola or 7-Up once in a while. Cola is useful for checking Clinitest tablets and reagent strips. See also URINE TESTS.

SOLUBLE INSULIN   See INSULIN.

SOLUTE   The dissolved substance in a solution.

SOLVENT   A liquid that dissolves another substance such as a sugar or salt without a chemical change taking place.

SOMATOMEDINS   A term that includes several distinct growth-hormone-dependent substances found in plasma, that have insulin-like activity. To be called a somatomedin, a plasma substance should be under control of a growth hormone, be insulin-like in action, and stimulate cell growth

226

in one or more of the body's tissues.

SOMATOSTATIN See RESEARCH.

SOMATOTROPIN An old name for GROWTH HORMONE (see).

SOMOGYI EFFECT See SLIDING-SCALE INSULIN COVERAGE.

SORBITOL A sugar alcohol. See SUGAR.

SORBITOL PATHWAY Polyol pathway. See Cataracts under EYESIGHT.

SORES See BED SORES; BOILS; BURNS; FOOT CARE; INFECTION AND INFLAMMATION; SKIN CARE.

SORE THROAT A condition caused by a number of factors, from a drip originating in the sinuses and irritating the back of the throat to a serious bacterial or viral infection. For temporary relief, gargle with salt water: boil 1 teaspoon of table salt in 1 pint of water for 10 minutes; cool to a comfortable temperature (very warm but not hot) before using. A sore throat accompanied by a feeling of sickness or malaise and an elevated temperature means you should check the urine four times a day and call your doctor. See also SICKNESS; THERMOMETER, CLINICAL; URINE TESTS.

SOUP The calorie and carbohydrate content of commercially made soups are available from the manufacturer on request. Cookbooks for diabetics* contain many recipes for making soup at home using food exchange lists. Soup in large amounts can be made and frozen into individual servings with the contents and calories on the label. Share recipes with friends. Sugar and salt substitutes can be used, but they are best added just before eating. See Salt Substitutes under SODIUM; Sugar Substitutes under SUGAR.

SPANISH DIABETIC DIET See FOOD EXCHANGES, Exchange Lists for Ethnic Foods.

SPECIFIC GRAVITY See URINE TESTS.

SPECIMEN A sample of urine, blood, stools, tissue, or any other substance to be used in tests.

SPHYGMOMANOMETER See BLOOD PRESSURE.

SPICES See CONDIMENTS.

*See Appendix B.

SPINAL CORD, SPINAL FLUID, SPINAL NERVES See CEREBROSPINAL FLUID; NERVOUS SYSTEM.

SPLIT-DOSES OF INSULIN Insulin given at two or more times a day. See INSULIN; RESEARCH.

SPONTANEOUS ABORTION See ABORTION; PREGNANCY AND CHILDBIRTH.

SPORTS See EXERCISE/SPORTS (includes a diet for exercise).

SRD State Registered Dietician. A trained dietician who has studied at college and who is licensed by the government. Most diabetic clinics will have such a dietitian available to talk to patients.

SRN State registered nurse. A trained nurse who has studied for 3 years. A state enrolled nurse (SEN) undergoes a shorter period of training. A district nurse (D/N) is usually an SRN, but who has received additional training on nursing in patients' own homes.

STABLE DIABETES See DIABETES, ADULT-ONSET.

STAGES OF DIABETES See Classification of Diabetes under DIABETES MELLITUS; PREGNANCY AND CHILDBIRTH.

STARCHES See CARBOHYDRATES; DIET; FOOD EXCHANGES, List 4; POLYSACCHARIDES.

STARVATION/STARVATION KETOSIS See FASTING; KETONE BODIES.

STASIS A slowing down or stoppage. Gastric stasis, or a delay in emptying of the contents of the stomach or the bowels, can be caused by diabetic neuropathy (which see).

STAT To be done right away – immediately. Abbreviation of *statim* (L)

STATISTICS ON DIABETES See DIABETES STATISTICS.

STEATORRHOEA See FAT DETERMINATION STOOL COLLECTION; LIPIDS.

STENOSIS The narrowing of a passagway, such as a blood vessel. See also HEART DISEASE.

STERILISATION OF SYRINGES AND NEEDLES See INSULIN SYRINGES AND THEIR CARE.

STEROIDS, STEROLS A group of fatlike (lipid) hormones made by the body in various glands. Progesterone, a female hormone, is an example of a steroid. See also ADRENAL

GLANDS; LIPIDS.

STOMACH PAIN When a person with diabetes has stomach pain, it indicates indigestion or stomach disease, or it can be a sign of diabetic ketoacidosis. If it persists, do not ignore it. Take your temperature, check the urine for glucose and acetone, and call the doctor. See also SICKNESS; THERMOMETER, CLINICAL; URINE TESTS.

Stomach and intestinal ulcers do not occur more often in the diabetic than in the general population. However, when they do occur, the control of diabetes becomes more difficult not only because of the necessary change in diet but also because of the added stress. See also STRESS.

STOOL TESTS See FAT DETERMINATION STOOL COLLECTION.

STORING INSULIN See DRUGS, STORAGE OF; TRAVELLING WITH DIABETES.

STRESS Hans Selye, MD, author of *Stress Without Distress* says that stress is the spice of life. People tend to think that stress in itself is bad, but actually it is one of the factors that can help people function at their best. It is bad when it causes worry, sleep loss, and anger.

Stress can be produced by both physical and emotional factors, such as sickness, injury, or infection, and pesonal conflict, frustration, fear, and loss. It affects both our mental and physical condition. Pregnancy and childbirth are stressful, as are certain other major life changes. It makes a big difference if you have someone to give you support during times of stress. Dr Roy Menninger, head of the Menninger Foundation, Topeka, Kansas, has studied the effects and causes of stress, and has been helping people to deal with it. What helps for one person, such as going for a swim, may not do it for another; he may have to go out and mow the lawn. What people need to do, Dr Menninger says, is to recognise when they are under stress and to pull back, look at the situation, and learn to deal with it. Diabetes can put a person in a situation in which he feels helpless – out of control. This can lead to depression, which is a very common way that people let stress dominate their lives. He says the danger signal that stress is more than a person can handle is a feeling of 'greyness' about the future. Menninger feels very strongly that the increase in serious illness in this country is the result of stress brought on about our rapidly changing ways of life. See also DIABETES MELLITUS, living with Diabetes.

Be sure to check the urine and acetone four times a day if you find yourself in a stressful situation, since glucose in the urine may be a clue that the body is stressed. Acetone in the urine is a further indication that control of your diabetes has slipped. Call the doctor so that he may help with the problem as necessary. See also SICKNESS; URINE TESTS.

STRESS TEST   See ELECTROCARDIOGRAM.

STROKE   See CEREBROVASCULAR ACCIDENT.

STUPOR   See COMA.

SUBCLINICAL DIABETES MELLITUS   See Classification of Diabetes under DIABETES MELLITUS.

SUBCUTANEOUS   Abbreviated sc, sub q, or H, subcutaneous means under the skin. See also HYPODERMIC; INSULIN INJECTIONS AND INJECTION SITES.

SUBSTITUTE DIET   See FOOD EXCHANGES.

SUCROSE   Table sugar. See SUGAR.

SUGAR   Most of the sugar we eat is table sugar, the sweet white or brown granules known technically as sucrose. The sources of this manufactured product are sugar-cane and sugar beets, and as sucrose they are chemically identical. However, sucrose is but one of several types of sugars, which are discussed below under Types of Sugars. For the person who must limit his intake of sugar – because of diabetes, or obesity, or both – it is important to know as much as possible about sugars so that he may successfully eliminate as much sugar as possible from his diet.

How the Body Uses Sugar   Sugar is a carbohydrate, and like all carbohydrates, it yields 4 calories per gram. To differentiate between sugar and other carbohydrates, such as starch, sugar is often referred to as a 'quick-acting carbohydrate'. Under normal conditions the calories supplied by sugar are used as energy; if not used immediately, they are stored in the liver and muscles as glycogen or are converted to fat. Simple or single sugars such as glucose and fructose do not have to be digested, and they enter the bloodstream almost immediately. Other more complex sugars are broken down

230

to single sugars quite rapidly; this allows them to be used, for example, in the treatment of low blood sugar (hypoglycaemia). Carbohydrates are converted 100 per cent by the body to glucose, and other foods can be converted to glucose in varying degrees (see GLUCOSE POTENTIAL OF FOODS). The problem confronting the diabetic is the rapidity with which all sugars enter the bloodstream and the resulting increase in blood glucose levels. The flow of blood carries the glucose to the cells, which need insulin in order that glucose may enter. Insulin is supplied either by the person's own pancreas or by injection. The nondiabetic can handle this increase in blood glucose, but the diabetic cannot, and the result is that abnormal amounts of glucose circulate in the blood. If the amount of glucose in the blood exceeds 9 to 10 mmol/L, glucose is spilled into the urine (see RENAL THRESHOLD), and the test for glucose in the urine is positive. The presence of very large amounts of glucose in the blood is a life-threatening situation called hyperglycaemia, and it can result in diabetic coma. See DIABETIC KETOACIDOSIS.

Recent research indicates that a large amount of glucose ingested at one time – such as that taken from an oral glucose tolerance test – acts in a different way from smaller amounts. It tends to remain in a glob in the stomach for a period of time until the stomach can rid itself of the load. Since this time may vary from person to person, this is one explanation of why so many different results are obtained from the oral glucose tolerance test (see BLOOD TESTS).

This phenomenon does not mean that it is therefore safe for the diabetic to eat a large amount of sugar at one time, because eventually all the sugar will be digested; and large amounts of sugar will require large amounts of insulin. On the other hand, it is extremely dangerous to increase the insulin dosage in anticipation of eating a large high-calorie meal, such as is served at Christmas or birthdays. In the nondiabetic, insulin is produced only as needed. For the diabetic, only a doctor can determine the amount of insulin needed, and he seeks to prescribe the smallest amount of insulin needed to cover the needs of the individual. Trouble results when the body is given either too much insulin

231

(hypoglycaemia) or too little (hyperglycaemia). Do not change your diet or your insulin dosage except on the doctor's approval.

A final note about sugar in the diet of the diabetic: The authors feel that the best solution for the diabetic is to re-educate the taste buds. Granted, this is hard to do, because people of the Western world have been brought up from infancy to include large amounts of sugar (and salt) in their diet, and the habit is deeply established. However, if one is motivated to achieve good control, weight loss, and good health, giving up a sweet tooth – like giving up cigarettes – is possible. In fact, eliminating sweets from the diet often results in the permanent loss of desire for them. Indications are, that after about six months of living without sweets, other than natural fruit, one tends to find them unpalatable; living without sweets is not difficult after that.

Types of Sugars There are several different types of sugars, all of which are known by the general term *saccharides*, which means sweet. Monosaccharides are simple or single sugars which do not have to be broken down or digested by the body; they include glucose and dextrose. (Dextrose is almost identical chemically to glucose and is used inter-changeably.) Glucose is found in most fruits and vegetables, and in honey. It is the form of sugar used by the body and measured in blood and urine tests. Fructose, or fruit sugar – also called levulose – is found in association with glucose in many fruits and vegetables and also in honey. Another single sugar, galactose, is seldom found free in nature but is part of lactose, or milk sugar. See BLOOD TESTS; PLASMA GLUCOSE; URINE TESTS.

The disaccharides, or double sugars, include sucrose, which is composed of the two single sugars glucose and fructose. It is found in most fruits and vegetables, and in honey. Maltose, or malt sugar, is made up of two glucose molecules; it is not found free in nature but is found in malted products such as beer and cereals. Lactose, or milk sugar, is also a disaccharide; it is produced only by mammals, and it is the only common sugar not found in plants. Broken down, lactose yields glucose and galactose.

Trisaccharides, not often discussed, include raffinose,

composed of three single sugars: glucose, fructose, and gālactose. It occurs in sugar beets, cottonseed meal, and molasses.

Polysaccharides, meaning 'many sugars', are complex sugars, such as starch, cellulose, and glycogen. They are also referred to as long-acting carbohydrates. Humans cannot digest cellulose, and glycogen is an internal product of the body. See CARBOHYDRATES.

Sugar in Food and Other Substances   The use of sugar in the Western world has increased at an alarming rate in the past century, with annual consumption averaging 115 to 125 pounds per person per year. It has been established that human beings have a taste for sweets, and processors of food use sugar to appeal to that taste. It is common knowledge that cakes, cookies, soft drinks, jams, and canned fruit contain large amounts of sugar, and many people are aware that most ready-to-eat cereals are made with sugar, but other foods may also contain large amounts of sugar, and a warning to read nutrition labels may not be sufficient to alert the diabetic. An examination of the labels on the packaged foods reveals that sugar is added to various kinds of food: canned corn, seasoned sweet peas, stewed tomatoes, canned soups, pork and beans, peanut butter, dehydrated soups, scalloped potatoes, stuffing mixes, barbecue sauce, gravy and chili mixes, canned ham, luncheon meats, and to some frankfurters, pickled herring, potato and marcaroni, many TV dinners, frozen pizza, frozen waffles, and canned Chinese food. Heinz ketchup is 28.9 per cent sugar, Shake'n Bake Barbecue mix is 50.9 per cent sugar, and Coffeemate nondairy creamer is 65.4 per cent sugar. If sugar is the number one ingredient, it is listed first on the label. However, it is not always listed as 'sugar' on labels, but may appear in the words glucose, dextrose, corn syrup, corn sweeteners, dextrin, and lactose. As a guide, look for words ending in 'ose'; they are likely to be sugars. Sugar alcohols end in 'ol' as do other alcohols. See Sugar Substitutes below.

Some medications such as liquid antibiotics and cough preparations often have sugar added. Be sure your pharmacist knows you have diabetes, and do not hesitate to ask him

233

if such medicines contain sugar. Over-the-counter drugs may contain sugar, so check the labels.

Sugar Substitutes Used widely to sweeten food, candy, gum, drugs, toothpaste, mouthwashes, and various drinks. They are divided into two main types: non-nutritive, without calories, and nutritive, with calories. Some sugar substitutes are mixtures of non-nutritive and nutritive ingredients. Non-nutritive sweeteners include cyclamate, now banned in the United States as a possible cancer-producing agent, and saccharin, also a suspected carcinogen. Saccharin comes in two forms: sodium saccharin and calcium saccharin. For those on a severely restricted sodium diet, calcium saccharin is recommended.

The amount of saccharin used in cooking affects the flavour of the dish. Too much tends to give a bitter taste, although the perception of this varies from person to person. Moreover, long cooking and high temperatures tend to reduce its sweetening power. Saccharin is best added toward the end of cooking, or after cooking, when possible.

New developments in artificial sweeteners include such low-calorie products as aspartame, a protein, not yet cleared for public use, and neo-DHC, made from citrus peelings.

Nutritive Sweeteners These are chiefly the sugar alcohols – carbohydrates yielding 4 calories per gram. They are metabolised more slowly than sugar, and are usually acceptable as a sugar substitute for the diabetic; however, the calories involved should be figured into the diet. Excessive intake of sugar alcohols can cause a positive urine test for sugar, and can cause diarrhoea. Sugar alcohols are sometimes used in combination with saccharin. Sorbitol is the most commonly used sugar alcohol, followed by mannitol and xylitol. Dulcitol and inositol are also in this group. Fructose, the single fruit sugar, is the sweetest of all the sugars, and is being used in the manner of artificial sweeteners by some food manufacturers. Do not use these products unless your doctor approves.

SUGAR ALCOHOLS See SUGAR.

SUGAR DIABETES See DIABETES MELLITUS.

SUGAR, FERMENTATION TEST FOR See URINE TESTS.

SUGAR-FREE Without sugar. The sugar alcohols, which are sugar substitutes, have calories. A pharmacist can advise you as to the sugar content of over-the-counter drugs. Liquid antibiotics usually contain sugar, as do cough syrups. See SUGAR.

SUGAR IN THE URINE (Glycosuria) See URINE TESTS.

SUGAR, QUALITATIVE/QUANTITATIVE TESTS See URINE TESTS.

SULPHONAMIDES Sulpha drugs. A group of drugs used to treat diseases caused by pathogenic bacteria. Some of the most widely prescribed are Bactrim and Septrin. Sulphonamides may react with the sulphonylureas (oral hypoglycaemic agents), intensifying their effect in further lowering the blood glucose. Sulphonamides are also photosensitive drugs and may increase the danger of sunburn.

SULPHONYLUREAS See ORAL HYPOGLYCAEMIC AGENTS.

SUMMER CAMPS See CAMPS.

SUNBURN See BURNS.

SURGERY The special problems of a person with diabetes who must undergo surgery are handled by the surgeons, usually in consultation with the patient's regular doctor. The surgery is usually performed early in the day, IV fluids are carefully selected, and the blood glucose is monitored closely. See RESEARCH.

SWEATING If you are sweating for no apparent reason, you may be suffering from low blood glucose. See HYPOGLYCAEMIC REACTIONS. An abnormal amount of sweat is called diaphoresis. An absence of sweating is anhidrosis.

SWEETS See SUGAR.

SWELLING See INFECTION AND INFLAMMATION; OEDEMA

SWIMMING See EXERCISE/SPORTS (includes a diet for exercise).

SYMPATHETIC NERVOUS SYSTEM See NERVOUS SYSTEM.

SYMPTOMS A change in or complaint of the body indicating sickness or disease. Disease such as diabetes can be present for some time without overt symptoms. See also DIABETES MELLITUS.

SYNCOPE Fainting.

SYNDROME A group of symptoms together indicating a particular problem or disease.

SYNTHESIS The making or building up of a substance. See also BIOSYNTHESIS; METABOLISM.

SYRINGES See INSULIN SYRINGES AND THEIR CARE.

SYRUPS See SUGAR.

SYSTEM In the body, a group of organs or structures that work together, such as the nervous system, digestive system, and respiratory system.

SYSTOLIC BLOOD PRESSURE See BLOOD PRESSURE.

T

TACHYCARDIA   A condition in which the heart beats at a rate of more than 120 beats a minute. Tachycardia may also be present when there is a significant increase in the heartbeat of a person who normally has a slow rate – below 60. It is an individual matter, and is discussed here only because a weak, rapid pulse is often present in diabetic ketoacidosis and other sicknesses.

TEA   Tea contains caffeine. Good substitutes are the herb teas that are found in supermarkets and health food stores. In hot weather try iced peppermint tea with a dash of sugar substitute; in cold weather, hot rose-hip tea, which is full of vitamin C.

TEENAGERS   See ADOLESCENCE; DIABETES MELLITUS, JUVENILE-ONSET.

TEETH   See MOUTH CARE.

TEMPERATURE   See DRUGS, STORAGE OF; FEVER; THERMOMETER, CLINICAL.

TENSION HEADACHES   See HEADACHES.

TEQUILA   See ALCOHOL.

TES-TAPE   See URINE TESTS.

TEST TUBES   See URINE TESTS.

TETANY   Severe muscle spasms. See METABOLIC ALKALOSIS.

THERAPEUTIC ABORTION   See ABORTION.

THERMOMETER, CLINICAL   An instrument used to take body temperature. Normal body temperature varies from person to person, but averages about 98.6° Fahrenheit, or 37° Celsius. Before taking a person's temperature, wipe the thermometer with alcohol, rinse in cold water, and shake down to below 95°F(34°C). Temperature can be taken orally, rectally, or in the armpit.

To take the temperature orally, use either an oral or a **rectal thermometer placed back under the tongue. For greatest accuracy, leave the thermometer in the mouth for 8** to 9 minutes, keeping the mouth closed. Breathing is done through the nose. If a person has been smoking, or having a hot or cold drink, wait at least 15 minutes before taking his temperature.

To take the temperature rectally, always use a rectal thermometer. Coat the bulb end with vaseline or some other lubricant. Place the patient on his side, and insert the thermometer gently and slowly into the rectum. Hold it in place with the hand for 3 minutes, remove, and wipe with a tissue to read. A correct rectal temperature cannot be taken if the thermometer is inserted into faeces, so be sure the bulb is against the side of the rectum. Rectal temperatures read one degree higher than oral temperatures; the average normal temperature of 99.6°F rectally is the same as 98.6°F orally.

For an axillary temperature place the bulb end of the thermometer in the centre of the armpit, close the arm snugly against the side of the body, and hold the thermometer in place for 10 minutes. Axillary temperatures read one degree lower than oral temperatures; a temperature of 100°F axillary is the same as 101° orally.

To clean a thermometer, wash it carefully in cold water with soap or detergent, then rinse it, dry it, shake it down, and replace it in its case. It is also a good idea to rinse it with alcohol.

With the use of the metric system becoming increasingly popular, a comparison table is included here and a conversion formula is included under the metric system (see next page).

THIRST See POLYDIPSIA.

THRESHOLD See RENAL THRESHOLD

THROMBOCYTES Platelets. See BLOOD; BLOOD TESTS.

THYMUS GLAND The human thymus is a flat organ consisting of two lobes or parts; it is located below the thyroid gland in the front of the chest just behind the breastbone. It is part of the lymph system. In the newborn, the thymus is large; it grows in childhood and reaches maximum size at the time of sexual maturity, after which time it gradually shrinks. The thymus is important in the development and

Comparison of Fahrenheit and Celsius temperatures:

CELSIUS	FAHRENHEIT
36.0	96.8
36.5	97.7
37.0	98.6
37.5	99.5
38.0	100.4
38.5	101.3
39.0	102.2
39.5	103.1
40.0	104.0
40.5	104.9
41.0	105.8
41.5	106.7

Note that both thermometers feature a scale that is 2/10° apart.

FAHRENHEIT

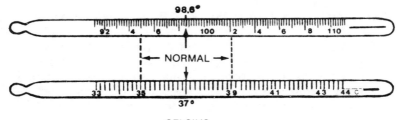

CELSIUS

function of the immune response, for it influences and programmes 'T' lymphocytes (white blood cells), which play an important role in protecting the individual against disease and infection. See also IMMUNE RESPONSE UNDER ALLERGY: LYMPH, LYMPHATICS; LYMPHOCYTES UNDER BLOOD; RESEARCH.

THYROID GLAND   A gland located in the neck in front of the windpipe (trachea) and just below the voice box (larynx). The fully developed human thyroid gland, seen from the front, looks like the 'wings of a butterfly', having two lobes or sections connected by a piece of tissue called the isthmus. The thyroid is controlled by the pituitary gland in the brain in a turn-on/turn-off cycle. Its hormones are necessary for growth, development, and sexual maturity, and regulate the basal metabolic rate, or the rate at which the body uses oxygen and produces heat. A change in metabolic rate could affect the control of diabetes, and this is one of the many organs doctors may need to test. See BASAL METABOLIC RATE; METABOLISM.

TIME ZONE CHANGES   See Jet Lag under TRAVELLING WITH DIABETES.

TINEA PEDIS   Athlete's foot; a fungus. See FEET, CARE OF; MICRO-ORGANISMS.

TINGLING   See DIABETIC NEUROPATHY: PARAESTHESIA.

TINNITUS   Ringing or other noise in the ears caused by drugs or disease. Aspirin, alcohol, and smoking can contribute to this disturbing problem. Diseases such as high blood pressure, arteriosclerosis, and endocrine disorders, including diabetes, can cause tinnitus. See Aspirin under SALICYLATES.

TIREDNESS   See FATIGUE.

TISSUE   A group of cells that are alike that unite to perform a particular function. Muscles, bone, skin, even the blood, are examples.

TOBACCO   *Tobacco·may be harmful to your health.* This statement can be found on the side of every cigarette package. Besides the probability that tobacco smoking increases the incidence of cancer and other lung diseases, there are other ways in which smoking can be harmful, When tobacco smoke is inhaled, carbon monoxide, a deadly gas, crowds out some of the oxygen the body needs. Smoking is also considered to be harmful to the blood vessels, to the heart, and especially to those who have retinopathy. Pregnant women, especially if diabetic, should not smoke. Cigarettes may burn the fingers; pipe and cigar smoke, although usually not inhaled, can cause sores and eventually cancer of mouth, lips, tongue and gums. Thus tobacco use in general compounds problems that may already be a factor in diabetes.

Chewing-tobacco has a sugar content between 10 and 25 per cent, with most brands contaning 15 to 20 per cent. Sugar can enter the system through the tissues inside the mouth.

TOENAILS See FEET, CARE OF.

TOLANASE See ORAL HYPOGLYCAEMIC AGENTS.

TOLAZAMIDE (Tolanase) See ORAL HYPOGLYCAEMIC AGENTS.

TOLBUTAMIDE (Rastinon or Orinase) See ORAL HYPO-GLYCAEMIC AGENTS.

TOLINASE Se ORAL HYPOGLYCAEMIC AGENTS.

TONIC See SOFT DRINKS.

TOOTHPASTE Most toothpastes are made with sugar substitutes. See SUGAR.

TOXAEMIA OF PREGNANCY A toxic or poisonous condition that is life-threatening to mother and baby. The early stage is called pre-eclampsia, progressing to eclampsia and toxaemia. More than the normal amount of amniotic fluid is present, a condition called hydramnios, or polyhydramnios, and defined as an amount of fluid in excess of 1,500 cc's. The first signs of toxaemia are weight gain, puffiness around the eyes and other signs of oedema, headache, and high blood pressure. Sugar and acetone will likely appear in the urine. It is extremely important that any of these warning signs be reported to the doctor *immediately*. See also AMNIOTIC FLUID; BLOOD PRESSURE; OEDEMA; PREGNANCY AND CHILDBIRTH.

TOXIC Poisonous.

TRADE NAME The name given to a product by the company that makes it.

TRAIN TRIPS   See TRAVELLING WITH DIABETES.

TRANSIENT, or TRANSITORY   Not lasting.

TRANSPLANTS   See RESEARCH.

TRANSPORT   Movement of nutrients through the bloodstream to the cells, and removal of waste products from the cells.

TRAUMA   Trauma is injury, sickness, or other stress – mental or physical. In the diabetic, trauma can cause diabetes to get out of control. See SICKNESS.

TRAVELLING WITH DIABETES   Travelling is stressful for anyone! However, the diabetic, with some extra planning, can travel anywhere in the world. For the diabetic interested in travelling, there is a useful book *The Peripatetic Diabetic*. It is an informative and amusing guide dealing with all kinds of problems of travelling from having a dinner on the town or at a friend's home to taking an around-the-world tour. The problems with the management of diabetes while travelling are somewhat dependent on whether the diabetes is controlled by diet alone or by diet supplemented with oral hypoglycaemic agents or with insulin. It is imperative that you always carry something to identify you as a diabetic, for instance, a Medic Alert bracelet or necklace. See MEDIC ALERT.

Eating at a local restaurant is easy if you have a good general knowledge of food exchanges. Dining at the home of a friend, especially if that friend does not know you have diabetes, can be handled by a phone call. After all, to pick at food at a great dinner without any explanation is rude and thoughtless. Perhaps all you would like to do is to skip the sour cream and gravy, go easy on the salad dressing, and eat a piece of fruit instead of pie à la mode for dessert. Trips by plane, ship, train, or bus are a little more complicated.

The following paragraphs are adapted from the *Meal Planning Booklet for Calorie Controlled and/or Diabetics' Diets*.**

Car Travel   If the driving time – to work or any other destination – is a half hour or less, adjustments in your diet will probably be unnecessary; however, if you are driving up to an hour or more it is wise to have a snack, especially at

**Printed with permission of Mary E. Wilson, RD, Clinical Dietitian, Kaiser-Permanente Medical Group, Fontana, California.

the end of the workday before starting on the drive home. The food should be taken from your evening meal. The following plan would be appropriate:

1 Bread exchange
1 Fat exchange
1 Meat exchange.

Put together, this would make half a sandwich.

In addition to having a snack before beginning a long drive, there are several other precautions to take:

1. Do not drink any alcholic beverage whatever before driving – alcohol and insulin together are a bad combination. (In addition, the slightest hint of alcohol on your breath could lead to a charge of drunken driving.)
2. Do not ever drive without have a source of sugar available (sugar cubes or a small can of orange juice are ideal). If you are simply a passenger in the car, you will probably not need to have a snack before driving but will need to have emergency sugar with you.

Bus Travel   If you ride a bus to and from work, you will want to have your emergency supply of sugar with you but will probably not need to make adjustments in your meal pattern because of the trip. When travelling for long distances (covering several meal-times), you will need to take enough sandwiches, fruit, and other foods to supply you for one or two meals. Bus travel for long distances is a difficult means of travel for all but the mildest of diabetics, since the time for stops can be altered by weather or other unpredictable conditions.

Rail Travel   For commuters, the same precautions as for bus travel to and from work should be followed. Travelling for long distances by rail is normally not difficult, because food is usually available on the train, but it is wise to take a sandwich and fruit with you in addition to your emergency sugar supply.

Travel by Ship   Food is normally readily available on board a ship, but seasickness can be a problem. If you become seasick, you should try to take orange juice, tea, milk, crackers, or dry toast immediately to 'cover' an insulin dose. See below for further suggestions to contend with motion sickness.

Air Travel Always check to see if a meal is to be served on the plane. If meals are not served, take a couple of sandwiches with you and carry your usual emergency supply of sugar. Some airlines serve meals for diabetics if they are ordered ahead of time. However, many seasoned travellers point out that meals are served at the convenience of the flight attendants rather than at normal mealtimes; in addition, long flights involve time-zone changes. Airplanes fly long-distance flights at altitudes between 35,000 and 45,000 feet, with cabin pressure controlled at the equivalence of 5,000 to 8,000 feet; which means that there is less oxygen in the air. A decrease in oxygen can result in a decrease in blood glucose. You may need to eat a few sweets (about 4), or drink some juice (½ cup orange juice or ¼ cup grape juice) if you feel a little lightheaded or headachy. Since alcohol tends to lower the blood glucose, especially on an empty stomach, it will be wise to abstain from alcoholic beverages. See also EXERCISE/SPORTS (includes a diet for exercise).

Motion Sickness Some people are prone to motion sickness, with nausea and even vomiting. It may be controlled in a number of ways; a cola drink or 7-Up is helpful for some; others may need a prescription drug – an antiemetic oral drug or suppository. Motion sickness is usually controlled with the drug Dramamine, available with a prescription. Again, consult with the doctor first. Dramamine can produce drowsiness to the point that can make driving unsafe.

Jet Lag Refers to the effect on the body caused by the changes in time zones that occur in travelling long distances by jet. For example, a flight from New York to London results in an 18-hour day, but the return trip is a 30-hour day. From the West Coast of the US the difference is even greater – subtract three hours going east and add three hours going west. This causes a distressing disturbance in the normal body rhythms, and particularly for the diabetic who is on a settled routine with diet and medication. Army researchers suggest adjusting to the trip in advance: A few days before leaving, eastbound travellers should go to bed an hour later than usual the third day in advance of the flight; 2 hours later the second day before the flight; and 3 hours later the day before the flight. Westbound travellers reverse the procedure. Discuss this with your doctor. For those on insulin, one approach the doctor may approve is to increase the usual insulin dosage by ⅓ and add an extra meal for every 8 hours added to the day; an example of this would be a flight from Europe to the West Coast. You would reverse the process on an eastbound trip, decreasing insulin by ⅓ and reducing the number of meals. However, *never* make changes in medication or diet except on the advice of your doctor.

Medication While Travelling   Unless you are an experienced traveller, you will also need to discuss with the doctor the amount and timing of the medication you take. For those who use insulin, there are a number of travel kits available commercially; Plastipak #8480 by Becton Dickinson is a good one. A home-made kit is easy to fashion from a Styrofoam packing box or sheets of this material, which can be purchased at hobby shops. Styrofoam is easily marked with a ruler and pencil, cut with a sharp knife, and glued together with white glue. Hold the box shut with a number of rubber bands while the glue sets. Rubber bands also serve well to keep the box together in transit. Arrange medication in an efficiently contrived space – include oral agents or insulin, other drugs, a few extra syringes, and some foil-wrapped alcohol swabs. Drug supplies of all kinds travel well when packed in the centre of a suitcase of clothing, which acts as both protection from breakage and an excellent insulator.

Carry extra medical supplies with you, and ask the doctor for copies of all your prescriptions. *Never carry all your drugs in one place.* If a suitcase is lost you may be in serious trouble. Divide drugs, syringes, swabs so that you have a supply on your person at all times. They can be carried in a purse or pocket, and in carry-on luggage, such as an over-the-shoulder tote. (Carry a spare pair of eyeglasses, too, if you wear prescription lenses.)

Customs   The following rules are taken from *Know Before You Go*, Office of Information and Publications: 'A traveller requiring medicines containing drugs or narcotics (i.e., cough medicines, diuretics (water pills), heart drugs, tranquillisers, sleeping pils, depressants, stimulants, etc) should:

1. Have all drugs, medicinal and similar products properly labelled.
2. Carry only such quantity as might normally be carried by an individual having some sort of health problem.
3. Have either a prescription or written statement from his/her personal physician that the medicines are being used under a doctor's direction and are necesary for the traveller's physical well-being while travelling.'

Travel Tips Luggage can be a trial while travelling, particularly since airlines seem to have a penchant for losing it. Take as little luggage as possible by planning a coordinated wardrobe made with drip-dry fabrics. A good rule is to lay out everything you plan to take and then cut the amount of clothing by half! A luggage dolly of the folding type is an energy saver, and can be taken on the plane as 'on board luggage'.

There are a number of organisations designed to help the traveller. The International Diabetes Federation (IDF) is a group that works to help diabetics all over the world. The International Luggage Registry (ILR) is a computer service. For an annual fee, members receive thirty-five stickers for their luggage that identify them as members of ILR. If luggage and other property is lost, the sticker supplies handling information. The stickers can be placed on eyeglass cases, tennis rackets, medical supplies, clothing, cameras, and, of course, luggage. Intermedic, Inc., lists English-speaking doctors in foreign countries who are qualified to care for diabetics. An annual membership is $5.00 a person, or $9.00 for the whole family.

Pamphlets for travellers include *A Guide to Accessibility of Airport Terminals*, a guide to airports and hotels with ramps for wheelchairs, available upon written request from Airport Operators' Council International; and *Air Travellers' Fly Rights* published by the Civil Aeronautics Board. You can write to E. R. Squibb & Sons for their free pamphlet *Vacationing with Diabetes, Not from Diabetes* and to the British Diabetic Association for *The Diabetic's Handbook*, which included information on holidays, travel, and jet lag. And the American Diabetes Association will send you *Travel Tips for Diabetics* for 15c and a self-addressed stamped envelope.

TREATMENT OF DIABETES   See DIABETES MELLITUS, Treatment.

TREMOR   See SHAKING.

TRIGLYCERIDES   See BLOOD TESTS; LIPIDS.

TRIPS   See TRAVELLING WITH DIABETES.

TRISACCHARIDES   See SUGAR.

TUBULE   A small tube or canal such as a nephron in the kidneys (see).

TUBERCULIN SYRINGES   See INSULIN SYINGES AND THEIR CARE.

TUMOURS   A swelling, or abnormal growth of tissue, that can be either cancerous or benign (noncancerous). A fairly uncommon type of tumour is an insulinoma, found in the beta cells of the pancreas. It is seldom cancerous, but the danger of this tumour is that it produces extra insulin, which in turn causes severe low blood glucose and results in damage to brain cells. Tumours of the alpha cells of the pancreas – called glucagonomas – are very rare.

Ultrasonography is being used effectively to detect tumours of the pancreas. For phaeochromocytoma, see ADRENAL GLANDS.

TWENTY-FOUR-HOUR URINE COLLECTION   See URINE TESTS.

TWO-DROP CLINITEST   See URINE TESTS.

TWO-HOUR POSTPRANDIAL TEST FOR SUGAR (2-hr PP) See BLOOD TESTS; POSTPRANDIAL.

U

U.G.D.P. STUDY   University Group Diabetes Programme. See ORAL HYPOGLYCAEMIC AGENTS.

ULCER   An open lesion on the skin or mucosa. Among the many types of ulcers are peptic ulcers in the stomach, and upper intestine, gastric ulcers in the stomach, and bed sores. A poor blood supply, injury, infection, or a combination of these can cause ulcers on the skin. The skin areas most likely to be affected are legs, feet, and toes. Check these areas every day. If you find a spot that does not appear to be healing normally, see a doctor. See also BED SORES; SKIN CARE.

ULTRALENTE INSULIN   See INSULIN.

ULTRASONOGRAPHY   Extremely high-frequency sound waves, much too high to be heard by the human ear, are used to probe the body in medical diagnosis. The procedure is painless, and up to this time there have been no reports of tissue damage or other harm to the patient. Ultrasound images can be printed on paper for reading and providing records in the prognosis of an illness or condition. Ultrasonography has been used, for example, to detect problems in pregnancy. See HEART DISEASE; PANCREAS.

UNCONSCIOUSNESS   See COMA.

UNILATERAL   On one side only, as on one side of the body.

UNIT OF INSULIN   See INSULIN.

UNIVERSITY GROUP DIABETES PROGRAMME   See ORAL HYPOGLYCAEMIC AGENTS.

UNMODIFIED INSULIN   Soluble insulin. See INSULIN.

UNSATURATED FATS   The same as monosaturated fats. See LIPIDS.

UNSWEETENED FOOD   Food without added sweeteners. Some foods are naturally sweet, and must be eaten in limited amounts by the diabetic, or by anyone who is on a reducing diet. Fresh fruits are naturally sweet, and the drying of fruit increases the percentage of sugar. Read the labels on packaged foods; many foods have sugar added before canning or freezing. See also DIETETIC FOOD; SUGAR.

UNTOWARD REACTION See SIDE EFFECTS.

URAEMIA See KIDNEY DISEASE.

UREA The chief end or waste product of protein use by the body (metabolism), which is excreted through the skin and the intestines, but mainly in the urine. When the kidneys function poorly, urea is not properly excreted, and collects in the blood. See also METABOLISM.

URETER One of two tubes or passageways carrying urine from the kidneys to the urinary bladder.

URETHRA A passageway for urine connecting the urinary bladder and the outside of the body. In the male, seminal fluid and sperm are also carried through this passageway.

URINARY BLADDER A hollow, stretchy organ that stores urine. When the bladder reaches a degree of fullness, around 200 to 300 cc's of urine, the need to void, or empty the bladder occurs. In disease, the urgency to void may vary tremendously. For example, in a bladder infection, a common symptom is urinary frequency, or the desire to void small amounts often. Also in infection, painful bladder spasms may be present, and the urine may burn on voiding. Diabetics are more susceptible to bladder infections, and any bladder infection endangers the entire urinary tract.

Urinary retention means that the bladder is not completely emptied on voiding, making infection even more likely. In the female, this may be caused by injury to the bladder during childbirth (correctable by surgery); in both male and female, it can be caused by nerve damage that impairs the elasticity of the bladder. Urine stasis, or failure of the urine to move out of the bladder after a large amount collects, can occur when the bladder stretches to hold a large amount or urine without the usual urgency signals to void. This is referred to as an atonic, a neurogenic, or a paralytic bladder. A pattern for voiding can prevent overfilling, in which the person can train himself to urinate by the clock. The bladder can also be palpated to judge its fullness. In examining yourself place the fingers of one hand on the lower abdomen and tap with the fingers of the other. By listening to the sound, you can determine the outline or edges of the bladder. A dull thud means you are over the bladder; a hollow sound means you have reached beyond the bladder to the area of the intestines. The inability to empty an overfull bladder requires medical attention. See CANDIDA ALBICANS; DIABETIC NEUROPATHY.

URINARY CATHETER See CATHETER.

URINARY FREQUENCY, URINARY RETENTION See URINARY BLADDER.

URINARY TRACT Includes the kidneys, ureters, urinary bladder (see), and urethra. See also URINE.

URINE A fluid waste product produced by the kidneys and stored in the urinary bladder. Any difficulty or pain on voiding should be reported to your doctor. Urine varies from an almost colourless fluid to dark yellow or brownish, depending on the relative amount of fluid in the body (hydration) and the kinds of foods eaten (beets turn the urine red). Haematuria (urine containing blood) may not change the colour of the urine; or the urine may look brownish or may look frankly like blood. Brownish urine may also be due to jaundice. Pneumaturia is foamy or bubbly urine caused by infectious bacteria that produce carbon dioxide gas.

URINE TESTS Urine as a waste product carries much information regarding the health of the body. There are many urine tests, ranging from very simple tests at home with tablets or dipsticks for the detection of glucose and acetone to complicated laboratory tests covering a period of several days in the diagnosis of suspected tumours or glandular disorders. Some tests relate to the detection and control of diabetes, and are discussed here.

Laboratory Tests The most commonly ordered laboratory test on urine is the urinalysis, or UA for short. The urine is tested for glucose, acetone, red blood cells, specific gravity, casts, pH, and bacteria. Most often a urine sample or specimen requested by the physician is brought into the doctor's surgery in a container supplied by the doctor or nurse. There are two general methods for catching the urine so that the information it provides is more reliable. One is the *midstream urine specimen* in which the patient is given a sterile container, asked to urinate a small amount that is not collected, stop the stream of urine, and void the remainder of the urine into the container; the other is the *clean catch urine specimen,* used when a culture is requested. The patient washes his/her genitalia with soap and water or with a cleaning solution provided by the nurse, and then proceeds as in the midstream collection. The female is further instructed in both collections to hold the labia (see GENITALIA) apart with one hand while voiding. It is also important that neither the inside of the container nor the lid is touched with the fingers, so that bacteria from the hands do not contaminate the specimen.

Tests for ketone bodies other than acetone are done in the laboratory when thought necessary.

Creatinine Clearance Test   A test for kidney function. Instructions may vary, but in general it is a collection of urine over a period of time, 24 hours or less, in which water intake of at least 100ml/hour should be maintained. Special diet instructions will precede the test. The urine should be refrigerated during the collection. The normal range for creatinine clearance is 100 to 140 ml/minute.

Twenty-Four-Hour Urine Collections   Can be made at home and taken to the laboratory for various tests. The procedure is standardised so that the patient is instructed to start the test in the morning. If 7.00 A.M. is specified as a starting time for the test, the bladder is emptied and this urine is not saved. All urine voided after this is saved and placed in a specially provided container. At 7.00 A.M. the next morning, the bladder is again emptied, but this urine is saved and is added to the collection. If an error is made during the collection, such as neglecting to add some of the urine, this must be reported; a new container must be obtained, and the collection restarted. Some containers are furnished with preservatives added so that the urine does not have to be refrigerated. Some collections must be refrigerated. If in doubt, refrigerate.

A urine collection may be analysed to determine the amount of glucose lost in the urine in a 24-hour period. Any amount over 5 per cent of the total daily calories is considered excessive. For the person on a 2,000-calorie diet, 5 per cent is 100 calories or 25 grams of glucose in 24 hours. A check may be made every 3 or 4 months if control of diabetes is difficult. At times, urine may be collected in aliquots, or fractional urine specimens, usually of 6 hours each, making four separate bottles necessary – each carefully labelled as to the time of collection. In this way, the time of day when glucose is being lost can be determined, and adjustments in insulin dosage and/or diet made.

Proteinuria, or the presence of protein in the urine, is usually in the form of albumin *(albuminuria)*, and a 24-hour collection of urine will best indicate this. It is a test for kidney function. It is also detected by various reagent strips, not described in this manual.

Home Tests   Urine tests for glucose and acetone may be done at home with dipsticks or tablets and are simple to perform. However urine testing at home is useful only as a rough guide to what is taking place in the blood. Those diabetics who have the tendency to hold large amounts of glucose in the blood before spilling it into the urine (high renal threshold), or whose blood glucose bounces back and forth, will get the least help from home urine tests. For tighter control, these diabetics may wish to investigate the use of Dextrostix for use with or without the Eyetone Reflectance Colorimeter.

The urine tests for glucose are usually taken before breakfast and before the evening meal. A first- or second-voided urine specimen may be used or both, depending on what is being checked. The first-voided specimen in the morning for those who have not voided in the night will have been in the bladder all night. Any sugar showing in this test will indicate that sugar has been spilled during the night, but will not indicate when. The second-voided specimen is obtained by drinking a glass of water after the first voiding, waiting ½ hour, and voiding again. This test is a better reflection of the blood glucose at this time.

To be meaningful, urine tests should provide information regarding the control of diabetes. This can be achieved only by a continuous set of records of test results, which will indicate such factors as whether blood glucose is being maintained at normal levels. It is therefore important to keep records of all tests. Clinilog is a handy way to do this. See also RECORDS.

Reagent Strips (or sticks) consist of specially treated paper supplied in a roll or attached to the end of a plastic stick. When dipped into urine according to instructions included in the package, chemicals impregnated in the paper react within a specified time for the detection of glucose, acetone, and other substances that may be present in the urine. Besides adhering strictly to time limits for the test, do not handle the area to be dipped into the urine; do not leave the test strips in a moist area (most bathrooms are too moist); keep the lid of containers tight; do not remove desiccant; and do not use test materials past the date printed on the side of the container. See DESICCANT.

It has been the custom in the past to report glucose in the urine in the following manner: If no glucose is detectable, the test is reported as negative; some tests next indicate a trace; then the tests are reported as 1+, 2+, 3+, or 4+. At other times the test may simply be reported as a certain colour. There are so many testing methods, each with a different plus value or colour reaction, that it is important to learn to report urine glucose results as a percentage. A chart is provided below to help with this reporting.

Tes-Tape (Eli Lilly Co.) It comes in a roll and is a popular way of testing for glucose in the urine because it is very sensitive and easy to carry. However, it tests only up to 2 per cent glucose. It is specific for glucose, and will not pick up lactose or other sugars, which therefore makes it useful for the nursing mother. Drugs that may give a false-positive test with Tes-Tape are vitamin C (ascorbic acid), levodopa, methyldopa (Aldomet), phenazopyridine (Pyridium), moderate-to-high doses of aspirin and other salicylates, and some drugs given in the treatment of cancer.

Clinistix (Ames Company) A reagent strip to test for glucose in the urine. It does not correlate with the percentage readings, and therefore is not recommended when a percentage report is desired. Drugs that may give false-negative tests are vitamin C (ascorbic acid), levodopa, phenazopyridine (Pyridium), aspirin, and other salicylates in moderate-

Concentration of Glucose in Urine in Percentage*

	.10% (1/10%)	.25% (1/4%)	.50% (1/2%)	.75% (3/4%)	1%	2%	3%	5%
Benedict's		+	++		+++	++++		or more
Clinitest 5-drop		trace	+	++	+++	++++		
Clinitest 2-drop		trace	+	++	++	+++	++++	+++++
Clinistix**	light +		medium ++			dark +++		
Test-Tape	+	++	+++			++++		
Diastix	trace	+	++		+++	++++		
Chemstrip G	trace	+	++		+++	++++		

*Spaces have been left blank when there are no colour codes for these concentrations.
**Does not correlate with percentages

to-high doses, tetracyclines given by injection or infusion, and drugs given in the treatment of cancer.

Diastix and Mega-Diastix (Ames Company) Reagent strips to test for glucose in urine. Mega-Diastix is an identical product to Diastix, made to a larger scale and with large-print instructions for those with visual impairment. If you are spilling moderate to large amounts of acetone, they may slow down the Diastix reaction, causing a lower reading; for example, a 1 per cent glucose might read as ½ per cent. If you are spilling a large amount of acetone, Ames recommends a re-check with Clinitest tablets. In any case, a large spill of acetone means something is wrong, so check with the doctor. Aspirin and vitamin C in large doses may cause false-negative tests with Diastix. See also SICKNESS.

Keto-Diastix (Ames Company) A reagent strip that measures both glucose and acetone in the urine. The test for acetone is read 15 seconds after dipping, and glucose is read 30 seconds after dipping in urine. A moderate-to-large amount of acetone may depress the colour development of the glucose test area, thus giving a lower reading for glucose. Drugs that may cause false-negative tests are large

254

doses of vitamin C (ascorbic acid) and false-positive tests with levodopa, phenazopyridine (Pyridium). Aspirin and other salicylates in high doses are listed as giving false-negative on glucose and false-positive on ketones.

Ketostix (Ames Company) A reagent strip to test for acetone in the urine. Drugs that may give a false-positive test result are levodopa, phenazopyridine (Pyridium), and aspirin and other salicylates in moderate to large doses.

To check for spoilage of Ames Company reagent test strip materials, prepare a solution of 1 teaspoon of regular Coca-Cola or 7-Up (not the diet type), mixed with ⅓ cup of water. Test as though testing for urine; the test result should read ¼ to ½ per cent glucose. If lower or higher results are obtained, replace the strips. Acetone is similarly tested using a solution of freshly opened Cutex or Revlon nail polish remover ¼ teaspoon mixed with ⅔ cup of water. Test as though testing for urine; the test should read small to moderate. Replace any test strips that give negative readings or turn colour different from the colour chart provided on the container.

Benedict's Solution The cheapest but least convenient test for glucose in the urine. Using a clean, dry test tube, and holding the medicine dropper pointing straight up and down, put 5 ml of Benedict's solution into the test tube. (This is about 1 teaspoon, or 15 to 16 drops.) To this, add 8 drops of urine and mix by gently shaking the test tube. Place in a bath of boiling water for 5 minutes. The colour chart supplied with the solution is converted to percentage in the table supplied in this section. Benedict's is a copper reduction test, is difficult to carry on trips, and is largely replaced by Clinitest.

Clinitest Reagent Tablets (Ames Company) Widely used to test for glucose in urine. They are not as sensitive to small amounts of glucose as Tes-Tape, but larger amounts of glucose can be measured with careful technique. There are some general warnings in the use of these tablets: They are very poisonous, very caustic, and should be kept out of the reach of children. Never use after the expiration date shown on the side of the package, and never use if the tablet shows signs of deterioration. Keep the bottle cap tightly screwed –

deterioration is usually caused by keeping the tablets in the bathroom where there is too much moisture. Excessive light and heat can also harm the tablets. A good tablet is off-white with a few light blue specks. A spoiled tablet has more specks, is darker blue, and may even become crumbly. Do not use chipped or broken tablets. A small testing kit, available at pharmacies, includes a plastic medicine dropper and a test tube. One test tube is not enough, however, because it is extremely important to use a dry test tube for each test. If a test is mis-started – the drops wrongly counted for example – start over again with a *dry* tube! Also, if a drop of water or urine hangs up inside the tube, it cannot be counted, and the test shoud be restarted. A 5-drop test may 'pass through the colours' (see below) and should be re-started as a 2-drop test – also with a dry test tube. A rack, easily made at home with dowels, will prove handy for storing a number of clean, dry test tubes. Similarly, the dropper should be throughly rinsed and shaken before switching from the measurement of water to urine. Ideally, a clean, dry dropper should be used each time a measure-ment is made. Both droppers and test tubes are inexpensive.

Do not drink the contents of the test tube! This caution is added here because people have actually ingested the contents of the test tube. As mentioned already, this is a poisonous mixture.

Drugs that affect Clinitests giving a false-positive reac-tion are vitamin C (ascorbic acid), Keflin/Keflex, chloramphenicol (Chloromycetin), levodopa, metaxalone (Skelaxin), methylodopa (Aldomet), nalidixic acid (Neg-Gram), phenazopyridine (Pyridium), probenecid (Be-nemid), aspirin in moderate to high doses, sulphonamides, tetracyclines (Achromycin, Panmycin, Sumycin), PASA (P-Aminosalicylic acid), Gantrisin injections, chloral hydrate (Noctec, Felsules). Keflin/Keflex is particularly noted for producing strange colours in tests, such as brownish black.

Five-Drop Test with Clinitest Reagent Tablets The most commonly used. A first- or second-voided urine specimen is collected as directed. Clean, fresh water should be available. (Plastic 1-ounce medicine cups are useful.) Holding a clean, dry test tube in one hand and at eye level, and holding the medicine dropper straight up and down, place 10 drops of water in the test tube. Squeeze the excess water out of the dropper and shake it, then take up some urine in the dropper and, using the same technique, carefully place 5 drops of urine into the water in the tube. Place the tube in a holder. You are now ready to put the Clinitest tablet into the water-urine mixture. The tablet should not be touched with your fingers. If you are using a bottle of tablets, shake one tablet into the bottle cap and carefully transfer the tablet into the test tube (and replace cap). Do not shake the test tube nor touch the tube at the bottom. The tablet produces a chemical reaction in which a great deal of heat is released. After 15 seconds, gently shake the tube and read the result as a colour. Translate the colour to a percentage from the chart at the beginning of this section. If there is a 'pass-through of colours' – that is, if the colour is orange momentarily and then changes to a muddy green-brown – there is greater than 2 per cent glucose. Take a clean dry tube and repeat the test using the 2-drop method.

Two-Drop Test with Clinitest Reagent Tablets Managed in the same way as the 5-drop test, except that 2 drops of urine and 10 drops of water are used. Obviously it is extremely important that a dry tube be used and that no drops hang up on the sides of the tube. This test shows up to 5 per cent glucose, and is the test recommended for persons who tend to spill glucose often. A kit with a special colour chart is available at the pharmacy for the 2-drop test.

One-Drop Test with Clinitest Reagent Tablets Done by using 1 drop of urine and 11 drops of water. Using the colour chart for the 2-drop test, bright orange indicates 10 per cent glucose. There is no kit for this test, and it is used mostly in 24-hour collections, or aliquots, when a large glucose spill is suspected.

Acetest Reagent Tablets (Ames Company) Used for testing the urine for acetone (see KETONE BODIES). These tablets should be kept in a dry, cool place away from excessive light. The normal colour of the tablet is white. A spoiled tablet is beige-tan brown. Do not touch the tablet with your hands, but instead pour it into the lid of the jar and then pour (place) the tablet on a paper towel. With a clean medicine dropper, place one drop of urine on the tablet, wait 30 seconds, and read the test by comparing the tablet colour change, if any, with the colour patches on the bottle label. If there is no colour change, the test is negative – there is no acetone present. If the urine does not absorb completely in 30 seconds, this means the tablet has been hardened by exposure to moisture and should not be used. Substances that give false-positive test results with Acetest are aspirin and other salicylates, levodopa and phenylketones.

URTICARIA ° See ITCHING.

USP Abbreviation for *Pharmacopeia of the United States of America* – a book of drugs that are approved by the Food and Drug Administration of the federal government. Substances are defined by source, type, physical and chemical properties, purity, and identity. Storage and dosage information is also given. See also DRUGS.

V

VACATIONS   See TRAVELLING WITH DIABETES.

VACCINE   A substance made in a laboratory and used to prevent or to treat some kinds of infectious diseases. Examples of these are measles and mumps (see both).

VAGINAL DISCHARGE   Secretions from the vagina. Abnormal secretion of the vagina is one of the most frequent reasons for which women seek medical attention. The vagina is a muscular passageway that functions as part of the sexual organs, and as the passageway through which a baby is born. It can be an area for infection, and increased or altered drainage should be brought to the attention of a doctor. See also CANDIDA ALBICANS; GENITALIA; INFECTION AND INFLAMMATION.

VARICOSE VEINS   Enlarged veins, usually in one or both legs, that can be very painful and unsightly. It is important to prevent injury and bleeding because of the danger of infection. Haemorrhoids (piles) are varicose veins of the rectal and anal areas. These conditions are correctable by surgery.

VASCULAR DISEASE   See BLOOD VESSEL DISEASE; HEART DISEASE.

VASCULAR SYSTEM   See BLOOD.

VEGETABLE JUICES   These are not included in the food exchange lists. The most common vegetable juice is tomato juice, which has about 40 calories per 6-ounce serving. For those who must limit sodium, salt-free juice is available at most supermarkets, or is readily made at home in a blender. Salt substitute should be added just before drinking. See Salt Substitutes under SODIUM.

VEGETABLE EXCHANGES   See Basic Four Food Groups under DIET; List 2 and Vegetarian Food Exchanges under FOOD EXCHANGES.

VEGETABLE PROTEIN   See PROTEIN.

VEGETARIAN FOOD EXCHANGES See FOOD EX-CHANGES, Vegetarian.

VEINS See BLOOD.

VENAPUNCTURE Puncture of a vein to draw blood (also called phlebotomy) or to inject or infuse drugs.

VIRAL INFECTION, VIRUSES See COXSACKIE B VIRUS; MEASLES; MICRO-ORGANISMS; MUMPS; RESEARCH.

VIROLOGY The study of viruses. See RESEARCH.

VISCERA, VISCERAL NERVES AND DISEASE The viscera are the organs inside the body, especially those of the abdomen. Nerve disease in this area can cause delayed emptying of the stomach, urinary bladder, and bowels, resulting in poor absorption of food. See also DIABETIC NEUROPATHY; NERVOUS SYSTEM.

VISION See BLINDNESS; EYESIGHT; RETINA, RETINO-PATHY.

VISUAL DISTURBANCES See EYESIGHT.

VITAL SIGNS The heart rate or pulse, the number of breaths (respirations) a minute, the body temperature, and the blood pressure are commonly called the vital signs.

VITAMINS A group of organic substances necessary for growth, healing, and general health. There is a great deal of disagreement about the amount of vitamins needed by the body. Vitamin B_{12} is needed to supplement a vegetarian diet; vitamin C is needed every day in some form; however, large doses of vitamin C can change urine test results. Your doctor is your best guide to the vitamins you need and the amount. See also FOOD EXCHANGES for some sources of various vitamins; URINE TESTS.

VITILIGO See SKIN DISEASES.

VITRECTOMY, VITREOUS FLUID See RETINA, RETINO-PATHY.

VITRO See IN VITRO.

VIVO See IN VIVO.

VODKA See ALCOHOL.

VOID To urinate. See URINE; URINARY BLADDER.

VOMITING See NAUSEA.

VULVA See GENITALIA.

W

WART A raised growth on the skin that is often rough. Because of the danger of infection, do not try to remove a wart by yourself. See the doctor.

WASTE PRODUCTS Substances no longer of use to the body. Examples are carbon dioxide, urea, salts, dead skin, undigested food, faeces, and water in the form of urine, sweat, and water vapour from the lungs. See also KREBS CYCLE.

WATER DIABETES See DIABETES INSIPIDUS.

WATER LOSS See DEHYDRATION; DIURESIS, DIURETICS; ELECTROLYTES.

WATER PILLS See DIURESIS, DIURETICS.

WAXY EXUDATES See RETINA, RETINOPATHY.

WEAKNESS A sudden feeling of weakness may be a sign of low blood glucose. If the onset of weakness is gradual, it may be due to a nervous system disease, or it may be from an inadequate diet, particularly from lack of iron. See also ANAEMIA; DIABETIC NEUROPATHY; HYPOGLY-CAEMIC REACTIONS.

WEIGHING FOOD See DIET.

WEIGHT: GAIN AND LOSS Although the term *overweight* is synonymously used with *obesity*, the terms are not the same. The obese person is defined as one who is 20 per cent or more over his ideal weight for his age, height, sex, and bone structure; an overweight person, according to these same standards, may weigh considerably more than his ideal weight, yet have little or no fat. This is found in heavy-boned, well-muscled men such as football players in good condition, and in persons who are genetically disposed to low body-fat. It is seldom seen in females, because females tend to have more body fat than males. Overweight is a word, however, that people fine less harsh than the words 'fat' and 'obese', and so it will continue to be used in that context.

Excess fat plays havoc with one's self-image, but the greatest damage is to health. Of particular concern to the diabetic is the fact that fat works against insulin; thus it is called an insulin antagonist. Obese people, whether they have diabetes or not, live shorter lives, have higher blood pressures, are sick more often, and are more likely to die suddenly than thin people. Fat is the biggest single problem in the adult diabetic. Most adult diabetics are obese, and about 80 per cent of adult diabetics could control their diabetes with weight loss and diet alone. It is estimated that the incidence of diabetes in the diabetes-prone individual is double for each 20 pounds of excess weight. There is some evidence that it benefits the adult diabetic to maintain a weight about 10 per cent below the ideal body weight.

How does one take off weight? The answer is easy: You must want to take off weight more than you want to eat too much, but unless you can fully accept the necessity and acquire the mental attitude, you will not take off weight nor keep it off. A reducing diet should be under the guidance of a doctor. Unhappily, less than 15 per cent of individuals who lose weight keep it off. Fad diets are dangerous and do not work; changes in life-style and eating habits are required. The problem of obesity in this country is so great that numerous studies are being conducted about it. It is known that it is harder for women to lose weight than for men and that it is harder to lose weight as one gets older; and finally, doctors have acknowleged that some people can eat almost nothing and still not lose weight. One of the reasons for this is that obese people tend to move around less than thin people, and the fatter they get, the less they move. In desperation, some doctors have hospitalised obese patients, putting them on a total fast in an effort to reduce poundage. See FASTING.

About 50 per cent of the body fat is just beneath the skin. Using skinfold measurements, a rough judgement can be made of how much body fat you have. Hold an arm straight out from your body. Under your upper arm, between elbow and arm pit, the skin and fat layer tends to droop. Gather this drooping area gently with the thumb and forefinger of the free hand; a woman aged 30-50 is obese if

DESIRABLE WEIGHTS

Weight in Pounds According to Frame (in Indoor Clothing)

	HEIGHT (with shoes on) 1-inch heels		SMALL FRAME	MEDIUM FRAME	LARGE FRAME
	Feet	Inches			
Men of	5	2	112-120	118-129	126-141
ages 25	5	3	115-123	121-133	129-144
and over	5	4	118-126	124-136	132-148
	5	5	121-129	127-139	135-152
	5	6	124-133	130-143	138-156
	5	7	128-137	134-147	142-161
	5	8	132-141	138-152	147-166
	5	9	136-145	142-156	151-170
	5	10	140-150	146-160	155-174
	5	11	144-154	150-165	159-179
	6	0	148-158	154-170	164-184
	6	1	152-162	158-175	168-189
	6	2	156-167	162-180	173-194
	6	3	160-171	167-185	178-199
	6	4	164-175	172-190	182-204

	HEIGHT (with shoes on) 2-inch heels		SMALL FRAME	MEDIUM FRAME	LARGE FRAME
	Feet	Inches			
Women of	4	10	92- 98	96-107	104-119
ages 25	4	11	94-101	98-110	106-122
and over	5	0	96-104	101-113	109-125
	5	1	99-107	104-116	112-128
	5	2	102-110	107-119	115-131
	5	3	105-113	110-122	118-134
	5	4	108-116	113-126	121-138
	5	5	111-119	116-130	125-142
	5	6	114-123	120-135	129-146
	5	7	118-127	124-139	133-150
	5	8	122-131	128-143	137-154
	5	9	126-135	132-147	141-158
	5	10	130-140	136-151	145-163
	5	11	134-144	140-155	149-168
	6	0	138-148	144-159	153-173

For girls between 18 and 25, subtract 1 pound for each year under 25.

*By courtesy of the Metropolitan Life Insurance Company.

the skinfold measures 30 millimetres, or a little over an inch; a man in the same age group is obese if the skinfold measures 23 millimetres, or just under an inch. Accurate measurements are made by a doctor with calipers. Skinfold measurements are also taken on stomach folds, and on the back below the shoulder blades.

Weight loss is a problem experienced by the young diabetic who is not getting enough to eat, or who is losing too many calories in the form of glucose in his urine. It can also be a problem with the adult insulin-dependent diabetic who is not controlled, and it is one of the symptoms in the diagnosis of the insulin-dependent diabetic, whatever his age.

WHISKY See ALCOHOL.

WHITE BLOOD CELLS See ALLERGY; BLOOD; BLOOD TESTS.

WHOLE BLOOD See BLOOD.

WINE See ALCOHOL.

WORK See EMPLOYMENT; EXERCISE/SPORTS (includes a diet for exercise).

XANTHELASMA   See SKIN DISEASES.
XANTHINES   See CAFFEINE.
XANTHOMATOSIS   See SKIN DISEASES.

YEASTS   See MICRO-ORGANISMS.
YOGURT   See FOOD EXCHANGES, List 1. Unflavoured yogurt can be used in place of sour cream for dressings and on potatoes. Since you should not use the sweetened fruit yogurts, substitute unflavoured yogurt and add fruit from the fruit exchanges (List 3) with or without sugar substitutes (see SUGAR). If you like, you can purée the fruit first in a blender, but do not put yogurt in a blender because it liquefies. This fruit and yogurt mixture is tasty on salads, or as a topping in place of syrup on pancakes or waffles.

Z

Z-TRACK INJECTION TECHNIQUE   See INSULIN INJEC-
TION AND INJECTION SITES.

Appendix A

ABBREVIATIONS AND SYMBOLS USED
BY THE MEDICAL AND NURSING PROFESSION

ac	before meals *(ante cibum)*
ACTH	adrenocorticotrophic hormone
ad lib	as desired
a.m.	morning
bid	twice a day *(bis in die)*
BMR	basal metabolic rate
BP or B/P	blood pressure
BS	blood sugar
c̄	with
C	Celsius (formerly centigrade)
caps	capsules
CBC	complete blood count
cc	cubic centimetre
CHF	congestive heart failure
CHO	carbohydrate
CNS	central nervous system
CO₂	carbon dioxide
CSF	cerebral spinal fluid
CVA	cerebral vascular accident
CVP	central venous pressure
dl	decilitre – ¹/₁₀ of a litre
Dx	diagnosis
EKG or ECG	electrocardiogram
EMG	electromyogram
F	Fahrenheit
FBC	Full blood count
FBS	fasting blood sugar
FBG	fasting blood glucose
GI	gastrointestinal

267

Gm (preferred), gm, g	gram
gr	grain
GTT	glucose tolerance test
GU	genitourinary
Gyn	gynaecology
Hb	haemoglobin
hr or h	hour
HHNK	hyperglycaemic hyperosmolar nonketotic coma
IM	intramuscular
IV	intravenous
IV GTT	intravenous glucose tolerance test
IVP	intravenous pyelogram
K	potassium
kg	kilogram
KUB	kidney, ureter, bladder
l or L	litre
Lab	laboratory
m or M	metre
mcg	microgram
MEq	milliequivalent
MI	myocardinal infarction
ml or mL	millilitre
mg or mgm	milligram
mm	millimetre
Na	sodium
OGTT	oral glucose tolerance test
O₂	oxygen
oz	ounce (also ʒ)
pc	after meals *(post cibal)*
p.m.	evening
po	by mouth – orally
prn	whenever necessary
qid	four times a day
RBC	red blood count
RBS	random blood sugar
RBG	random blood glucose
RDS	respiratory distress syndrome
Rx	treatment (prescription)

sc	subcutaneously
stat	immediately – right now
tid	three times a day *(ter in die)*
TPR	temperature, pulse, respiration
WBC	white blood count
Wt	weight

Appendix B

COOKBOOKS

BENNETT, MARGARET. *The Peripatetic Diabetic*. The guide to good health and good times for those who have diabetes. New York: Hawthorn Books, Inc., 1969.

BOWEN, ANGELA. *The Diabetic Gourmet*. New York: Harper & Row, 1970.

DONAHUE, VIRGINIA. *Diabetic Cooking Made Easy*. Revised and enlarged edition. Minneapolis, Minn.: Burgess Publishing Co., 1973.

GIBBONS, EUELL AND JOE. *Feast on a Diabetic Diet*. New York: David McKay Co., 1969.

GORMICAN, ANNETTE. *Controlling Diabetes with Diet*. Springfield, Ill.: Charles C. Thomas, 1976.

JONES, JEANNE. *The Calculating Cook: A Gourmet Cookbook for Diabetics and Dieters*. San Francisco: 101 Productions, 1972.

———— . *Diet for a Happy Heart*. New York: Charles Scribner's Sons, 1975.

KAPLAN, DOROTHY. *The Comprehensive Diabetic Cookbook*. New York: Frederick Fell, Inc., 1972.

REVELL, DOROTHY TOMPKINS. *Gourmet Recipes for Diabetics*. Springfield, Ill.: Charles C. Thomas, 1971.

WALDO, MYRA. *The Low Salt, Low Cholesterol Cookbook*. New York: G.P. Putnam's Sons, 1972.

WEST, BETTY M. *Diabetic Menus, Meals and Recipes*. Garden City,

N.Y.: Doubleday and Co., 1978
WOMEN'S AUXILIARY OF THE LOMA LINDA SCHOOL OF MEDICINE
ALUMNI ASSOCIATION. *An Apple a Day – Vegetarian Cookbook.*
Loma Linda, Calif.: Loma Linda School of Medicine, 1967.

Appendix C

SUGGESTED READING

BENNETT, MARGARET. *The Peripatetic Diabetic.* The guide to good health and good times for those who have diabetes. New York: Hawthorn Books, Inc., 1969.

BIERMANN, JUNE, and TOOHEY, BARBARA. *The Diabetes Question and Answer Book.* Los Angeles: Sherbourne Press, Inc., 1974.

———— . *The Diabetes Sports and Exercise Book.* Los Angeles: Sherbourne Press, Inc., 1977.

DANOWSKI, T.S. *Diabetes as a Way of Life.* New York: Coward-McCann and Geoghegan, Inc., 1974.

DOLGER, HENRY, and SEEMAN, BERNARD. *How to Live with Diabetes.* Rev. ed. New York: Pyramid Books, 1977.

DUNCAN, GARFIELD G. *A Modern Pilgrim's Progress.* 2nd ed. (Also available in Spanish). Philadelphia and London: W. B. Saunders Co., 1967.

FISCHER, ALFRED E., and HORSTMANN, DOROTHEA L. *A Handbook for the Young Diabetic.* New York: Stratton Foundation, Inc., 1972.

GRABER, ALAN, and CHRISTMAN, BARBARA G. *Diabetes and Pregnancy.* Edited by Patricia C. Pearson. Nashville, Tenn.: Vanderbilt University Press, 1973.

ROGERS, FLOYD L.; LEVERTON, RUTH M.; and HERVERT, J. WILLIAM. *Your Diabetes and How to Live with It.* 3rd ed. Lincoln: University of Nebraska Press, 1961. University Microfilms.

SCHMITT, GEORGE F. *Diabetes for Diabetics.* Williamsport, Pa.: Bro-Dart Books, Inc., 1968.

SINDONI, ANTHONY M., JR. *The Diabetic's Handbook: How to Work*

With Your Doctor – Treatment by Diet, Insulin and Oral Medication. 2nd ed. New York: John Wiley & Sons, 1959.

TALBERT, BILLY (WILLIAM F.), with SHARNIK, JOHN. *Playing for Life.* Boston: Little, Brown and Co., 1959.

TRAVIS, LUTHER B. *An Instructional Aid on Juvenile Diabetes Mellitus.* 5th ed. (Also available in Spanish). Galveston, Tex.: University of Texas Medical Branch, 1978.

YUDKIN, JOHN. *Sweet and Dangerous.* New York: Bantam Books, 1973.

Appendix D

EMERGENCIES

An emergency is an unforeseen situation calling for immediate action. A medical emergency is life-threatening and can occur in anyone's life. In the life of a diabetic, medical emergencies must be handled by the medical profession, with skilled nursing care and access to a laboratory for frequent tests.

The major medical emergencies in diabetes occur as the result of alterations in the blood glucose level; these change the chemistry of the body and may alter the level of consciousness (see COMA). High blood glucose levels are present in DIABETIC KETOACIDOSIS and HYPERGLYCAEMIC HYPEROSMOLAR NONKETOTIC COMA (HHNK) – (see both). (See also LACTIC ACIDOSIS.) Low blood glucose (hypoglycaemia) is a medical emergency that should first be treated at home by giving the individual sugar of some kind (see HYPOGLYCAEMIA and HYPOGLYCAEMIC REACTIONS), because over a prolonged period low glucose can damage brain cells. *Always treat unconsciousness as low blood glucose if in doubt as to the cause.*

Unfortunately few doctors have time to educate and inform their patients properly, and they are not always available

271

when you need help. If an emergency exists and your doctor is not available, use the facilities of a hospital. Some hospitals are staffed 24 hours a day with specially trained doctors. Find out which hospitals in your area are so staffed and place their phone numbers in a quickly accessible place – such as the front cover of your phone book or the wall beside your phone – along with other emergency numbers. Dialing 999 will connect you with the police, fire department, and ambulance services. They will give you help over the phone and, if necessary, dispatch an emergency vehicle to your home. Instruct all members of your household in the importance of this emergency number, including children, who are also capable of saving lives. Make a practice drill to show the children in your home how to dial the number and what to say over the phone. This is as important as a fire drill.

Injuries and other trauma to the body and mental state can be potential emergencies; for example, a cut on one's foot is a potential infection site for all, but the diabetic is more prone to infection. Don't go barefoot, and don't neglect any cut. If a cut, burn, or abrasion does not heal quickly, see your doctor. You will find many potential medical problems in the text listed in alphabetical order, from ALLERGY to WART. Also, be sure to read and discuss SICKNESS with your doctor. If you are going on a trip, read TRAVELLING WITH DIABETES.

Errors in medication, especially when made continuously over a period of time, are responsible for some emergencies, but if you simply forget to take one insulin injection, do not get upset. Check with your doctor, who will probably tell you to take about two-thirds your regular dose with a small amount of soluble insulin added. If you take too much insulin by accident, eat some extra carbohydrate in the form of Dextrosol, soft drink or orange juice, and increase the bread allowance in your next snack or meal. The effects of taking too many or too few pills (see ORAL HYPOGLYCAEMIC AGENTS) may be felt only over a long period of time, because their effect on the body is longer than that of insulin. Watch for a delayed reaction the next day. In the event of medication errors with either insulin or pills, do frequent urine tests for glucose to help you and your doctor decide on the proper course of action. NOTE: Every diabetic should have a vial of soluble insulin on hand in the refrigerator. The family should know it is there. Syringes should also be available, and you and your family should know how to give an insulin injection (see INSULIN INJECTION AND INJECTION SITES).

Diabetes must not be treated lightly, but at the same time it is unwise to live in a state of panic, worrying when the least little thing goes wrong. Emotional support from family, friends, and local diabetes groups, as well as membership of the British Diabetic Association, are all helpful in times of stress. With education and the proper care, the diabetic can lead a long, active, and happy life.

Directory

ASSOCIATION OF BRITISH
PHARMACEUTICAL
INDUSTRY
162 Regent Street
London W1
(01) 734-0961

ASSOCIATION OF BRITISH
TRAVEL AGENTS
55 Newman Street
London W1
(01) 637-2444

BRITISH AIRPORTS
AUTHORITY
2 Buckingham Gate
London SW1
(01) 834-6621

BRITISH AIRWAYS
(IMMUNISATION AND
MEDICAL)
Victoria Terminal
London W1
(01) 834-2323

BRITISH ASSOCIATION
FOR DISABILITY AND
REHABILITATION
25 Mortimer Street
London W1
(01) 637-5400

BRITISH DENTAL
ASSOCIATION
63 Wimpole Street
London W1
(01) 935-0875

BRITISH DIABETIC
ASSOCIATION
10 Queen Anne Street
London W1
(01) 323-1531

BRITISH DIETETIC
ASSOCIATION
305 Daimler House
Paradise Street
Birmingham 1
(021) 643-5483

BRITISH HEART
FOUNDATION
57 Gloucester Place
London W1
(01) 935-0185

BRITISH HOMOEOPATHIC
ASSOCIATION
27a Devonshire Street
London W1
(01) 935-2163

BRITISH INSURANCE
ASSOCIATION
Aldermary House
Queen Street
London EC4
(01) 248-4477

BRITISH MEDICAL
ASSOCIATION
Tavistock Square
London WC1
(01) 387-4499

BRITISH NURSING
ASSOCIATION
(Private nurses organisation)
470 Oxford Street
London W1
(01) 723-8055

BRITISH RED CROSS
SOCIETY
9 Grosvenor Crescent
London SW1
(01) 235-5454

BRITISH WIRELESS
FOR THE BLIND
224 Great Portland Street
London W1
(01) 388-1266

DEPARTMENT OF HEALTH
AND SOCIAL SECURITY
Alexander Fleming House
Elephant and Castle
London SE1
(01) 407-5522

DEPARTMENT OF TRADE
(For enquiries about
availability of medicines
overseas)
1 Victoria Street
London SW1
(01) 215-7877

HYPOGUARD LIMITED
49 Grimston Land
Trimley, Ipswich
Suffolk IP10 0SA
(03942) 75689

HEALTH SERVICE
COMMISSIONER
(THE OMBUDSMAN)
157 Blackfriars Road
London SE1
(01) 633-9216

HM CUSTOMS AND EXCISE
(For enquiries about taking
medicines through customs)
(01) 283-8911

HM STATIONERY OFFICE
(Official publications
relating to diabetes
and nutrition)
Atlantic House
Holborn Viaduct
London EC1
(01) 928-1321

KIDNEY RESEARCH FUND
184b Station Road
Harrow
(01) 863-4469

MEDISTRON LIMITED
Alpine Works
Oak Road
Crawley, Sussex
(0293) 513535

METRICATION BOARD
22 Kingsway
London WC2
(01) 242-6828

PASSPORT OFFICE
(Telephone numbers vary
with your surname)
Petty France
London SW1

PHARMACEUTICAL
SOCIETY OF GREAT BRITAIN
1 Lambeth High Street
London SE1
(01) 735-9141

ROYAL COLLEGE OF
NURSING
Henrietta Place
London W1
(01) 580-2646

ROYAL NATIONAL
INSTITUTE FOR THE BLIND
224 Great Portland Street
London W1
(01) 388-1266

SOCIETY OF CHIROPODISTS
8 Wimpole Street
London W1
(01) 580-3227

Index

NOTE: Main entries on specific subjects are not listed in this index. They may be found, in alphabetical order, in the text. However, when main entries appear elsewhere without cross-reference, they are indexed.

Abdominal aorta, 157
Abdominal pain, 107
  in diabetic ketoacidosis, 62
  hyperglycaemic hyperosmolar
    nonketotic coma and, 128
  pancreatitis and, 190
Abrasion, 76
Acid-base balance, 157
ACTH (adenocorticotropic hormone),
  18
ADH (antidiuretic hormone), 56
Age, glucose tolerance and, 118
Albumin, 34, 73, 163
Albumin test, 36
Albuminuria, 19
Alcohol (alcoholic beverages) 88, 107
  hypoglycaemia and, 131
  oral hypoglycaemic agents, and, 184
Alcoholism, 190, 215
  acute, 159
Alcohol rub, 29
Ale, 107
Alfalfa sprouts, 107
Alka-Seltzer, 223
Allergy to insulin, 138-39
Almonds, 99
Amino acids, 69
Anger, 60
Angiography, 190
Ankles, charcot joints in, 47
Ant bites, 30
Antibiotics, 192
  for influenza, 137

Antibodies, in autoimmunity, 26
Antidiuretic hormone (ADH), 56
Anuria, 155
Anxiety, 111, 129
Appetite, lack of, 24, 190
Apple cider, 92
Apples, 88, 92
Applesauce, 92
Apricots, 92
Arrowroot crackers, 95
Arteriosclerosis, 42
Artichokes, 88, 194
Asparagus, 91
Aspirin, 159, 186
Atherosclerosis, 39, 207
Athletes, 76
Atromid-S, 186
Audio and visual aids, 83
Autoantibodies, 26
Avocado, 99
Avoidance of reality, 111-12

Back pain, 190
Bacon, 99, 225
Bacon fat, 99
Bactrim, 235
Bagels, 94
Bananas, 92, 194-95
Barbecue sauce, 233
Barley, 94
B-D Plastipak syringes, 148-49
Beans, 22, 43, 96
Bedwetting, 75

277

Beef, 97, 98
Beer, 107
Beet greens, 91
Beets, 91
Behavioral research in diabetes, 210
Belching, 136
Benemid, 186
Bicarbonate, 74
Bilirubin test, 36
Biscuits, 95
Blackberries, 88, 93
Bladder. *See* Urinary bladder
Blood clotting, 33
Blood poisoning, 27
Blood pressure, 128, 214
  in pregnancy, 197
Blood vessel complications of diabetes,
  207-8
Blood vessel disease, 184-85
  degeneration in, 54
Blood volume, measurement of, 47
Blueberries, 88, 93
B lymphocytes, 33
BMR, 27
Body fat, 138
  See also Obesity
Bones, charcot joints and, 47
Books for the visually handicapped, 83
Bouillon, 109
Brain neuroglycopaenia and, 180
Brain damage, hypoglycaemic
  reactions and, 131
Bran flakes, 94
Bread crumbs, 94
Breads, 22, 94
Breathing, hypoventilation and, 133
Broccoli, 88, 91
Bronze diabetes, 120
Broth, 109
  instant vegetable, 225

Brussels sprouts, 88, 91
Buckwheat groats, 87
Burgundy wine, 19
Burns, 114
Buttermilk, 90
Butazolidin, 186
Butternut squash, 95

Cabbage, 88, 91
Caecum, 151
Cake, 108
Calcium, 89
Candy, 108
Cantaloupes, 92, 93
Capon, 98
Carbohydrates
  digestion of, 69
  for hypoglycaemic reactions, 131
Carrots, 88, 91
Cauliflower, 88, 91
Causes of diabetes, research on, 205-6
Cavities, 177
Celery, 88, 91, 224
Celery flakes, seed, or salt, 225
Cell membrane, 208
Cellulose, 194
Cereals, 180, 224
  ready-to-eat (with sugar), 108, 233
Chablis wine, 19
Chards, 91
Cheddar cheese, 98
Cherries, 93
Chicken, 97
Chick-peas, 161
Chicory, 92
Children, 60, 186
  congenital defects in, 50
  hepatomegaly (enlarged liver) in, 164
  measles vaccine for, 168
  summer camps for, 42-3

Chili mixes, 233
Chili sauce, 225
Chinese cabbage, 92
Chinese food, canned, 233
Chloramphenicol, 186
Chloride, 74
Cholesterol, 96, 186
  electrophoresis of, 73
Cholesterol test, 36
Cirrhosis of the liver, 114, 164
Citrus fruits, 92
Clams, 97
Coca-Cola (Coke), 132, 226
  See also Cola drinks; Soft drinks
Coffee, 109
Coffeemate nondairy creamer, 108, 233
Cola drinks, 42, 226
  See also Coca-Cola
Cold cuts, 98
Collard greens, 91
Colon, 151
Coma, 155, 159, 208
  hypoglycaemic, 130, 131
Complete Blood Count (CBC), 36
Condoms, 51
Consciousness, levels of, 49
Constipation, 87
Cookies, 108
Corn, 87, 95
  canned, 233
Corn bread, 95
Corn chips, 226
Corned beef, 97, 98, 225
Cornmeal, 95
Corn muffin, 95
Coronary heart disease, 121
Coronary thrombosis, 122
Cortisone-Primed Oral Glucose
  Tolerance Test, 37
Cottage Cheese, 97

Cough preparations, 233
Courgettes, 91
C-peptide, 138
Crab, 97
Crackers, 95, 226
Cranberries, 93
Cream, 99
Cream cheese, 99
Creamer, nondairy, 233
Cucumber, 91
Cures for diabetes, research on, 206
Cysts, acne, 17

Dandelion, 91
Dates, 93
Dehydration, 74, 128, 155
  diaphoresis and, 64
  diarrhoea and, 64
  in lactic acidosis, 159
Depression, 60
  stress and, 229
Dextrostix, 197
Diabetes, juvenile-onset: blood vessel
  disease in, 39
Diabetes mellitus
  as bihormonal disease, 29, 114
  hemochromatosis and, 120
  Diabetic Diet Guide, 89
Diabetic ketoacidosis, 74, 155
  abdominal pain and, 15
  acetonuria in, 16
  ataxia in, 25
  breathing and, 19, 40
  coma and, 49
  dehydration in, 54
  glucagon levels and, 114
  glucose as osmotic diuretic in, 59
Diabetic neuropathy, 216
  constipation and, 50
  dysuria in, 62

foot drop and, 108
Dialysis, 156
Diaphragm, 51
Diarrhoea, 74, 107, 190
Diastolic blood pressure, 35
Diet
  amino acids in, 22
  for exercise, 77-8
  after heart attack, 122
  iron in, 23
  in pregnancy, 196-97
  low-sodium, 223-26
  reducing, 65, 261-62
  during sickness, 218-19
Digestion, incomplete or poor, 136
Diuretics, 192
Doctor, choosing a, 61
Dosage of insulin. *See* Insulin dosage
Doughnuts, 108
Duck, 98
Duodenum, 151

Eggplant, 91
Eggs, 180
Ejaculation, retrograde, 63
Elbows, xanthomatosis on, 221
Electrolytes
  diabetic ketoacidosis and loss of, 62
  diarrhoea and loss of, 64
Endive, 92
English muffins, 94
Epsom salts, 86
Erection, 216
Eructation, 136
Escarole, 92
Ethanol, 19
Exchange Lists for Meal Planning, 88-9
Exercise
  ECG taken during, 73
  laxative effect of, 160

leg pain after, 160-61
Exocrine glands, 113
Eyelids, drooping of the, 200
Eyes, dehydration and, 54
Eyesight, 214

Farmer's cheese, 98
Fast, seventy-two-hour, 216
Fasting Blood Glucose, 37
Fats, digestion of, 69
Fatty acids, 69, 84
Fever, 74, 128, 215
  indigestion and, 136
Fibre, 87-8
Fibrinogen, 33
Figs, 93
Fish, 88, 97, 180
Folic acid, 89, 91-4
Food, labelling, 182
Frankfurter roll, 94
Frankfurters, 98, 225, 233
French dressing, 99
Fruits, 180, 224

Gardening, 120
Garlic, 194
Garlic salt, 225
Gastric stasis, 228
Gastric surgery, reactive
  hypoglycaemia after, 130
Gelatine, unsweetened, 109
Globulins, 33
Gloves, 31
Glucagon, for hypoglycaemic
  reactions, 124
Glucose
  alcohol and, 19-20
  amino acids and, 22
  bacteriuria and, 27
  chromium and metabolism of, 48

depression and, 55
diabetic ketoacidosis and, 62
diabetic neuropathy and, 63
digestion and, 68-9
diuretics and, 69
emotional changes and, 74
fasting and, 84
glucagon and, 114
glucocorticoids and, 116
glycogen and, 118
headaches and, 112-13
hyperglycaemia and, 127-28
hypoglycaemia and, 129-32
kidney disease and, 155
in lactic acidosis, 159
neuroglycopaenia and, 180
niacin and, 180
in pregnancy and childbirth, 195-96
in urine, 119, 169
Glycogen, 22, 194
Glycosuria, 119
Goose, 98
Grains, 43
    See also Cereals
Grapefruit, 92, 93
Grapefruit juice, 92, 93
Grape juice, 93
Grapes, 93
Gravies, 225
Gravy mixes, 233
Green peppers, 88, 91
Greens, 91
Gums, 58

Haematocrit, 32
Ham, 97, 98, 225
    canned, 233
Hamburger, 88
Hamburger buns, 84
Hammer-toes, 87

Hand, Dupuytren's contracture of, 72
Hearing problems, 214
Heart
    circulation of the blood and, 34
    in diabetic ketoacidosis, 62
Heart disease, 19, 169, 196
Heart failure, 159
Heatstroke, 74, 215
Heinz ketchup, 233
Herb teas, 237
Herring, pickled, 233
Histamine, 33
Histidine, 22
Honey, 108
Honeydews, 92, 93
Horseradish, 225
Hose, 86
Hydrocortisone, 52
Hyperglycaemic hyperosmolar
        nonketotic coma, 49, 74, 114
    dehydration in, 54
    glucose as osmotic diuretic in, 69
Hypertension (high blood pressure),
    types and causes, 19, 47, 169
Hyperventilation, 159
Hypoglycaemia
    aggressiveness and, 19
    coma and, 49
    in infants, 198
    snacks and, 101
Hypoglycaemic reaction
    drowsiness in, 70
    glucagon as emergency treatment
        for, 114
    intramuscular injection and, 151
    oral hypoglycaemic agents and,
        184-85
    sickness and, 218
    sports and exercise and, 77

INDEX

Ileum, 151
Infants, hypoglycaemia in, 198
    See also Children
Infection
    lymphatic system and, 166
    glucocorticoids and, 116
Insulin
    bovine, 40
    expiration date of, 71, 140
    storage of, 71
Insulin dosage, 139
    in adolescence, 18
    hypoglycaemia and, 130, 131
    inactivity and, 135
    sickness and, 28, 217
    sports and exercise and, 77
Insulin injection and injection
        sites, 129
Insulinoma, 128
Iron in diet, 23, 94, 96
Ischaemia, 28
Isoleucine, 22
Italian dressing, 99

Jam, 108
Jejunum, 151
Jelly, 108
Jerusalem artichokes, 194
Jet-spray automatic syringes, 149
Joslin Clinic, 56
Joslin Diabetes Foundation, 89
Juices, 132
    apple, 92
    grape, 93
    grapefruit, 92, 93
    orange, 92, 93
    pineapple, 93
    prune, 93
    tomato, 91
    vegetable, 91, 259

Kaiser-Permanente Diet Manual, 218
Kale, 91
Keflex, 220
Keflin, 220
Ketchup (catsup), 50, 225, 233
Ketosis, 167
Kidney disease, 19, 159, 196
Kidneys, microangiopathy and, 39
Kidney transplants, 206

Labelling, 182
Lactic acidosis, 74
    coma and, 49
    dehydration in, 54
Lamb, 97, 98
Lard, 99
Lecithin/sphingomyelin (L/S) ratio, 197
Lemon, 109
Lentils, 43, 95, 161
Lettuce, 88, 92
Leucine, 22
Leukocytes (white blood cells),
        differential count of, 68
Libraries, 83
Liver (food), 88, 96, 97, 186
Liver (human)
    gluconeogenesis in, 116
    glycogenesis in, 118
    haemochromatosis and, 120
    inflammation of the, 123
Liver cirrhosis, 114, 164
Liver disease, 159
Lobster, 97
Luncheon meats, 233
Lymph nodes, 165-66
Lymphocytes, 165
    allergic reactions and, 21
Lysine, 22

Macaroni, 95
Mackerel, 97
Macroangiopathy, 207
Macular oedema, 211
Magazines for visually handicapped
    people, 83
Magnesium, 96
Mangoes, 92, 93
Manometer, 46
Marmalade, 108
Massage for tension headache, 121
Mazzoth, 95
Meat, 88, 180
Meat extracts and tenderisers, 224, 225
Medijector automatic syringes, 149
Melons, 93
Methionine, 22
Microangiopathy, 27, 39, 207
    in juvenile-onset diabetes, 58
Milk
    condensed, 108
    goat's, 119
    for insomnia, 137
    instant nonfat dry, 137
    skim, 137
Molasses, 108
Monoject syringes, 148
Mozzarella, 98
Muscle, wasting of, 23, 151
Muffin, 94
Mushrooms, 91
Mustard, 108
    prepared, 225
Mustard greens, 91

Nausea, 107, 136, 190, 214
    in diabetic ketoacidosis, 62
Nectarines, 92, 93
Neufchâtel, 98
Nicotinamide, 180

Nicotinic acid, 186
Nitroglycerin (NTG), 122
NPH insulin, 101
Noodles, 95
Noradrenaline, 18
Nuts, 88, 226

Obesity, 114, 128, 138
    fatty liver in, 164
    reactive hypoglycaemia and, 130
    See also Diet, reducing
Oestrogens, 50, 127
Oils, vegetable, 98, 99
Okra, 88, 91
Oliguria, 128, 155
Olives, 99, 225
Onions, 91, 194
Oral hypoglycaemic agents, 192
    alcohol and, 20
    aspirin and, 214
    bedtime snacks and, 101
    hypoglycaemia and, 131
    pregnancy and, 196
    during sickness, 28
Orange juice, 92, 93
Oranges, 92, 93
Orgasmic response, 21
Osmolality, 188
Osmolarity, 188
Osmotic pressure, 188
Ovaries, 177
Oyster crackers, 95
Oysters, 96, 97

Pain-killing drugs, 178
Pancake, 96
Pancreas, 189
    hyperinsulinism and, 128
    inflammation of, 85
Pancreatic carcinoma (or cancer), 85, 190

hyperglycaemic hyperosmolar
  nonketotic coma caused by, 128
Pancreatitis, 20, 114
Papayas, 92, 93
Paraesthesia
  blisters and, 31
  burns and, 41
  in feet, 86
  sheetburn and, 28-29
Parmesan, 98
Parotid glands, 177
Parsley, 92
Parsley flakes, 226
Parsnips, 88, 95
Pasta, 95
Pastrami, 22
Peaches, 88, 92, 93
Peanut butter, 96, 98, 226, 233
Peanuts, 99
Pears, 88, 93
Peas, 88, 95, 96
Pecans, 99
Peppermint tea, 237
Peripatetic Diabetic, The, 242
Persimmons, 92, 93
Phaeochromocytoma, 18
Pheasant, 97
Phenformin HC1, 159
Phenylalanine, 22
Photocoagulation, 209
Pickles, 109, 225
Pie, 108
Pigmentary cirrhosis, 120
Pineapple, 93
Pineapple juice, 93
Pituitary ablation, 213
Pizza, frozen, 233
Plastipak #8480, 245
Platelet count, 36
Plums, 93

Poisoning, 215
Polydipsia in juvenile-onset
  diabetes, 57
Polyneuropathy, 47
Polyuria in juvenile-onset diabetes, 57
Popcorn, 95
Pork, 97, 98
Pork and beans, 233
Pork insulin, 139
Port, 19
Potassium, 74, 92, 94, 96
  diabetic ketoacidosis and loss of, 62
Potato chips, 226
Potatoes, 43, 88
  scalloped, 233
Poultry, 97, 98
Pregnancy, German measles and, 168
Preserves, 108
Pretzels, 95, 226
Protein, 97
  nitrogen balance and, 180
Protein synthesis, 119
Prune juice, 93
Prunes, 93
Psychosocial research in diabetes, 210
Puberty, 17-18
Pulse, 214
Pumice stone, 86
Pumpernickel bread, 94
Pumpkin, 94, 95
Pustules, acne, 17

Radishes, 88, 92
Rail travel, 243
Raisin bread, 94
Raisins, 93
Raspberries, 93
Red cell count, 36
Reflex, Achilles tendon, 16
Relishes, 50, 226

Retina, microangiopathy and, 39
Retinal detachment, 212
Retinopathy, 211
Rhine wine, 19
Rhubarb, 91, 109
Rice, 22, 43, 94, 180
    brown, 87
Ricotta, 98
Rose-hip tea, 237
Rosé wine, 19
Rubbing alcohol, 20, 29
Rutabagas, 91
Rye bread, 94
Rye wafers, 95

Salad dressing, 99
Salicylates, 159
Salicylism, 186
Salmon, 97, 225
Salt pork, 99
Sardines, 97, 226
Sauerkraut, 91, 226
Sausage, 225
Sauterne, 20
Scallops, 97
Scalp wounds, 31
7-Up, 132, 226
Sherry, 19
Ship, travel by, 243
Shrimp, 97
Sickness, glucose tolerance and, 118
Sleep, 137
    hypoglycaemic reactions and, 132
Snacks, 101
Socks, 86
Soda crackers, 95
Sodium, 223
Sodium salicylate, 214
Soft drinks (with sugar), 42, 108
Somatic neuropathy, 63

Somatostatin, 133
Sorghum, 108
Soups
    canned, 225, 233
    dehydrated, 233
    dried, 225
Soybeans, 161
Soy sauce, 226
Spaghetti, 95
Spinach, 91
Steroids, anabolic, 186
Stomach pain, 136
Storage of drugs, 71
Strawberries, 93
Stress, 229
    glucose tolerance and, 118
    headaches caused by, 121
    menopause and, 169
Stress ECG, 73
String beans, 91
Stuffing mixes, 233
Stupor, 159
Sugar, 108
    in chewing tobacco, 241
    exercise and, 77
    in urine, 169
Sulpha drugs, 186
Sulphonamides, casts in urine and, 45
Sun, sensitivity to the, 192
Sunburn, sulphonamides and, 235
Swabs, alcohol, 20
Swallowing
    hypoglycaemic reactions and, 131
    through windpipe, 25
Sweating, 221
    fever and, 87
    upon waking, 132
Sweet peas, 233
Syrups, 108
Systolic blood pressure, 35

INDEX

Systolic hypertension, 35

Tabasco sauce, 109
Tanderil, 186
Tangerine, 93
Tea, 109
  peppermint, 237
  rose-hip, 237
Tenting, 54
Thiamin, 94
Thirst in diabetic ketoacidosis, 62
Threonine, 22
Throat, sore, 227
Thrush, 43
Tingling, 50
  charcot joints and, 47
T lymphocytes, 33
Tomatoes, 91
  stewed, 233
Tomato juice, 91
Tomato paste and sauce, 226
Tongue, dry, 54
Tortilla, 94
Trace minerals, 176
Tranquillisers, 192
Triglycerides, electrophoresis of, 73
Tryptophan, 22
Tubal ligation, 51
Tuna, 97, 225
Turkey, 96, 97
Turnip greens, 91
Turnips, 88, 91
TV dinners, 233
Twins, identical, 134

Ultrasonography, 190, 197, 241
Unconsciousness, 155
U100 insulin, 140
Urinalysis, 250
Urinary bladder, cystogram of, 53

Urinary incontinence, 75
Urine
  albumin in, 19
  bacteria in, 27
  blood in, 120
  diabetes insipidus and, 56
  glucose in, 169
Urine tests during pregnancy, 197

Vaginal infections, 169
Valine, 22
Vasectomy, 51
Veal, 97, 98
Vegetable broth, instant, 225
Vegetable juice, 91, 259
Vegetable oils, 98, 99
Vegetables, 43, 88, 180, 224
Venules, 34
Vinegar, 109
Visceral neuropathy, 63
Visual and audio aids, 83
Visual handicapped persons
  audio and visual aids for, 83
  magazines for, 83
Vitamin A, 89, 91, 92
Vitamin B-complex, 89, 96, 186
Vitamin B_{12}, 89, 96, 260
Vitamin C, 91, 92, 260
Vitamin D, 90, 162
Vitamin E, 162
Vitamin K, 162
Vitreous haemorrhage, 211-12
Vomiting, 74, 107, 136, 159, 214

Waffles, 96
  frozen, 233
Walking, pain after, 160
Walnuts, 99
Washing, 27
  feet, 86

Wasp stings, 30
Wasting
  interosseous, 151
  of muscle, 23
Watercress, 92
Water loss
  in diabetes insipidus, 56
  fever and, 87
  See also Dehydration
Weakness, 167
Weight gain
  in menopause, 169
  in pregnancy, 169
Weight loss
  fasting for, 84
  See also Diet, reducing
Wheat germ, 95
White blood cells, differential count of,
    36
White cell count, 36
White cell differential count, 36
Whole wheat bread, 94
Wine, 19, 107
Worcestershire sauce, 226
Wounds, bleeding from, 31

X-rays, 24
  intravenous pyelogram, 151
Xylitol, 234

Yams, 88

Zinc, 96